Essential Skills

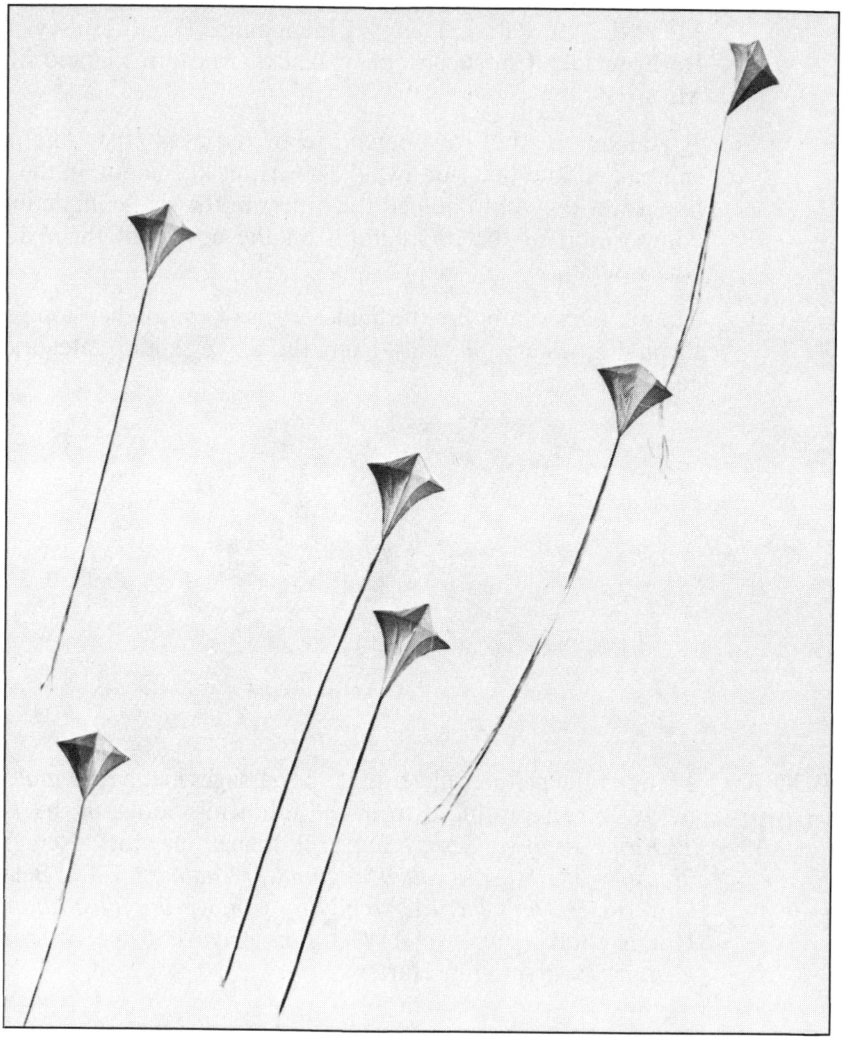

Revised Edition

About the Cover

The breeze was fresh this bright day in May, and gaily-colored kites appeared like spring swallows, darting across the blue sky over Rhode Island's Narragansett Bay. Photographer Tony Botelho was there to capture on film the kite-flights of Christy Menard, Art Pelosi, Danny Champagne, Peggy Hulsey, John Rathjen, Jack Christie, Stephen Jencks, Marion Alig and Megen Mills.

A salute to the rowboaters who retrieved the "diamond-spinnaker" kite that got away! The errant kite shook in the wind like a wet dog and rejoined the others in the sky, completing the composition of the photograph on the covers of the *Essential Skills Series*.

The six kites symbolize the higher levels of comprehension gained through mastery of skills from the six essential categories of comprehension.

About the Illustrations

Many of the pictures illustrating the passages in the *Essential Skills Series* were reproduced from the following books in the *Dover Pictorial Archive Series*, Dover Publications, Inc., New York: *Treasury of Art Nouveau, Design and Ornament*, Carol Belanger Grafton; *Harter's Picture Archive for Collage and Illustration*, Jim Harter; and *Animals: A Pictorial Archive from Nineteenth-Century Sources*, Jim Harter.

Other illustrations are by Howard Lewis and Thomas Ewing Malloy.

Essential Skills Series

Essential Skills Book 13

Walter Pauk, Ph.D.
Director, Reading Research Center
Cornell University

Revised Edition

Jamestown Publishers
Providence, Rhode Island
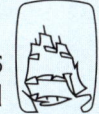

Essential Skills Series
No. 313, Book 13

Copyright © 1982 by Jamestown Publishers, Inc.

All rights reserved. The contents of this book are protected by the United States Copyright Law. It is illegal to copy or reproduce any pages or parts of any pages. Address all inquiries to Editor, Jamestown Publishers, Post Office Box 6743, Providence, Rhode Island 02940.

Cover Design by Deborah Hulsey Christie, adapted from the Original Design by Stephen R. Anthony

Text Design by Deborah Hulsey Christie

Printed in the United States AL

85 86 87 88 9 8 7 6 5 4

ISBN 0-89061-232-3

Preface

Practice Makes Perfect

Why do some students shoot baskets over and over again and others skate and reskate the same routine? These beginners know that practice makes perfect. Not only do beginners know this, but pros do too. For what other reason do they work at baseball and football week after week before the opening dates?

Value of Practice

The pros know the value of practice, but they also know the value of something else. They know that practice without *instruction* and *guidance* does not automatically lead to improvement. That's why they have the best coaches that money can buy.

And so it is with developing the skills of reading. There must be the right kind of practicing and the right kind of coaching.

First, a word about practice. In this book the right kind of practice is provided by twenty-five highly interesting and carefully selected passages. Here is material enough on which to grow and keep growing.

Value of Coaching

Now about coaching! Good coaching takes the form of instruction and guidance. In this book the instruction is straightforward and uncomplicated. It puts you directly on the right track, and better still, you are kept on the right track by two unusual systems of guidance. The first system is the uniquely designed, six-way question format which makes sure that every ounce of practice is directed toward improvement. Nothing is wasted!

Diagnostic Chart

The second system of guidance is the Diagnostic Chart. This chart is no ordinary gimmick. In truth, it provides the most dignified form of diagnosis and guidance yet devised. It provides instantaneous and continuous diagnosis and gentle but certain self-guidance. It yields information directly to the student. This form of self-guidance leads to the goal of all education: the goal of self-teaching.

Acknowledgments

Now, I want to make some acknowledgments, especially to the students who were the guinea pigs. Afterwards I told them so, but they said, "We didn't mind even then. And now that it is over, we're all the happier because we know how much we've learned." But what the students did not know was how much I learned from them. For this I thank them all, class after class.

I direct especial thanks to Linda Browning, Anita DuBose, and Karen Duddy for handling the almost countless number of selections, writing and refining the questions and making sure that the series kept moving: all, a most demanding task.

Finally, I am most grateful to authors, editors and publishers who have generously given permission to quote and reprint in this book from works written and published by them. The books quoted in the text and used as sources of reading extracts are listed in the back of the book.

Walter Pauk

Contents

To the Instructor **8**

To the Student **11**

    Understanding the Six Essential Skills **11**
    Answering the Main Idea Question **17**
    Getting the Most Out of This Book **19**

Passages and Questions **23**

Answer Key **100**

Diagnostic Chart **102**

Progress Graph **103**

Classroom Management System **106**

To the Instructor

Selection of Passages

All of us believe in this truism: to learn to read, a person must read. But, placing a book in front of a student won't automatically promote reading.

This last sentence brings up another truism: you can lead a horse to water, but you can't make it drink. To tempt a horse, the water must be clear, cool and clean.

To tempt the student, the passages must be genuinely fascinating. Knowing this, we packed each book with twenty-five "I can't put the book down" type of passages.

Each passage had to meet at least the following criteria: *high interest level, appropriate readability level* and *factual accuracy of contents*. High interest was assured by choosing passages from popular magazines that appeal to a wide range of readers. The readability level of each passage was assessed by applying Dr. Edward B. Fry's *Formula for Estimating Readability,* thus enabling the arrangement of passages on a single grade level within each book. The factual accuracy of the passages is high because they were written by professional writers whose works are recognized and respected.

The Great Value of Questions

Dr. Mortimer J. Adler says that the overall secret for improving one's reading can be boiled down to knowing how to keep awake while reading. He means more than keeping one's eyes open. He means keeping one's mind open and active.

One sure-fire way to do this is to keep trying to answer questions while reading. Questions not only keep one's mind awake, but also keep the mind active, not letting it get flabby. Here's a good story that makes the same point.

> To keep their fish alive for the fresh-fish markets, the owners of fishing boats used a water-filled floating tank. The fish remained alive all right, but they were never firm, always flabby. One captain, however, always brought back firm, fresh, active fish. His fish always received a higher price.

One day he revealed his secret: "You see," he said, "for every hundred herrings I put into my tank, I put in one catfish. It is true that the catfish eat five or six of the herrings on the trip back to port, but the catfish keep the rest alert and constantly active. That's why my herring arrive in beautiful condition."

The work of the catfish, in this book, is done by the six essential questions (subject matter, supporting details, conclusion, clarifying devices, vocabulary in context, and main idea). These questions keep the minds of students alert, active and in beautiful condition.

The main idea questions in this book are not the usual multiple-choice variety. Given four statements, the students are asked to recognize the main idea of the passage. They also tell why each of the other three does not express the main idea; the students identify one statement as too narrow, one as too broad and one as merely a detail.

By asking these six types of questions in each passage, students quickly learn to read with a questioning and anticipating attitude. This attitude, necessary for high comprehension, is easily transferred to other material such as the textbook.

The Diagnostic Chart

Those who used the first edition of these books had high praise for the Diagnostic Chart. In sum, this is what they said.

> The Diagnostic Chart is truly ingenious because it is, in fact, a self-diagnosing instrument. The Chart instantly, simply and continually shows students their strengths and weaknesses.

Here is how the Chart works. The six questions for each passage are always in the same order. For example, the question designed to teach the skill of making *conclusions* is always in the number three position, and the question designed to teach the skill of identifying *clarifying devices* is always in the number four position, and so forth. This innovation of keeping the questions in order sets the stage for the smooth functioning of the Chart.

The Chart works automatically when the letters of the answers are placed in the spaces on the Chart. Even after completing one passage, the Chart will reveal the type or types of questions answered correctly as well as the types answered incorrectly. But more important, the Chart will identify the types of questions missed consistently. More persuasive identification is possible after three or more passages have been completed. By then, a pattern can be observed. For example, if the answers to question number three (making conclusions) are incorrect for all three passages, or on three out of four, then this weakness shows up automatically.

Once a weakness is revealed, instruct the students to take the following steps: First, turn back to the instructional pages to study the section in which the topic is discussed. Second, go back to read again the questions in that particular category that were missed; then, with the correct answers in mind, read the entire passage again, trying to see how the author developed the answers to the questions. Third, on succeeding passages, put forth extra effort to answer correctly the questions in that particular category. Fourth, if the difficulty still persists, arrange for a conference with the instructor.

To the Student

Understanding the Six Essential Skills

What reading skills does a person have to know to gain meaning from written facts? To get meaning, most people would have to know at least six essential skills. They would have to know how to learn to glean the subject matter, to grasp main ideas, to relate supporting details to main ideas and sub-ideas, to draw conclusions, to recognize clarifying devices, and to unlock the meaning of words. Let's take a closer look at these skills.

Concentration/ Subject Matter

There is no problem that I hear more frequently than, "I can't concentrate!" Fortunately, there's a sure, fast cure. There is no better magic for gaining concentration while reading than this one: after reading the first few lines of a passage, softly ask yourself this question: "What is this passage about?" In other words, "What's the general subject matter?"

If you don't ask this question, here's what will generally happen: your eyes will move across the lines of print while your mind is still entertaining the lingering thoughts of a previous conversation or daydream.

If you ask the question, however, you will almost always arrive at an answer, thus capturing concentration. Let's see whether or not this technique works. Here are the first lines of a passage:

> Wood ducks are the most beautiful ducks in North America. Once they were rare. Now — if you have sharp eyes and can keep quiet — you might see them in almost any woodland, along streams and ponds.

Obviously, you can say with a great degree of assurance that the author is going to talk about the wood duck. Now that your mind is on the trail, the chances are great it will follow the author's ideas paragraph after paragraph, thereby *concentrating* on the development of the subject matter.

Let's try the technique again. Here are a few lines from another passage:

> Of all the little animals in the world, the Columbian ground squirrel is one of the liveliest and friendliest. It is nicknamed "picket pin" because it sits as stiff and straight as a stake on the ground.

Again, you probably experienced no trouble at all zeroing in on the subject matter: the Columbian ground squirrel.

Main Idea Once the general subject matter has been quickly ascertained, it is easier for the mind to grapple with the next question: What is the author's main idea? What point is the author trying to get across?

With such questions in mind, you will be surprised at how often an answer pops up. When no questions are asked, it seems that everything is on the same level — nothing stands out.

Let us peruse another short excerpt, this time for the main idea.

> Wood ducks never nest on the ground as most ducks do, but in a big hole in a tree. Trees with big holes in them are hard to find.

Since you don't have the full passage to read, may I make this comment: The main point that the author is making is that with the scarcity of old, dead trees with holes in them, we will have fewer and fewer wood ducks.

Thus, we see that by asking questions, reading becomes a two-way street. When we talk with the author, the author seems to come to life. Reading then becomes an exciting and enjoyable experience.

Supporting Details Are we interested in details? Of course we are! In longer passages, main ideas and sub-ideas are the bones, the skeleton of the passages. The details are the flesh which gives passages completeness, fullness and life.

Details are used almost entirely to support the main idea and sub-ideas. Consequently, the term *supporting details* is appropriate. These supporting details come in various forms, but the most common forms are: examples, definitions, comparisons and contrasts, repetitions and descriptions.

The author of "The Wood Duck" has supplied us with enough information so that we know the passage is about wood ducks. Next, the author made sure that we understood the point that without "trees with big holes in them" the wood duck will not nest; thus, there would be fewer wood ducks.

Having gotten us interested in this unique problem, the author then supplied details on how we could provide "trees with big holes in them." The author *described* how we could build a wood duck nesting box. Here's the excerpt:

> Why don't you and your parents put up a wood duck nesting box right now? It would be about two feet high and ten inches square. Make the entry hole about four inches in diameter. Use rough lumber on the inside so the ducklings can climb up the sides to the hole. Put wood shavings in the bottom in which the duck will lay her eggs. To keep her eggs warm, she covers them with her own feathers. If you don't have a tree near the water, you'll need a post. Place the box ten to thirty feet high.

You can see in the above example how important details are in telling a story. Details enable the reader to visualize what's going on, how to do something, how to take action, and so forth.

In any passage of length, there will be some or many sub-ideas. It is important to be sufficiently wary so as not to mistake a sub-idea for a main idea. One way to distinguish between the two is as follows: The main idea pertains to the entire passage, whereas the sub-idea pertains only to a portion of it. Notice that in the following example the sub-idea is about the food that wood ducks eat. The entire passage is *not* about food, so it is *not* the main idea. In most cases you will see that a sub-idea takes the space of one paragraph.

The main purpose for including the following excerpts is to show how the author clusters and organizes supporting details around the relatively minor sub-ideas that are stated in topic sentences. In other words, a sub-idea is the nucleus that holds a body of details together.

> Wood ducks like to eat acorns and all kinds of nuts. Their stomachs (or gizzards) have such powerful muscles that they can break the hardest nuts, some that you could barely crack with a hammer! Wood ducks like berries, duck weed and insects. But best of all they like to eat spiders — that's ice cream to them.

The author, after adding to the passage a brief but detailed description of some food that wood ducks eat, continues to describe how the newly hatched ducklings get down to the ground from some dizzy heights. Here are more details clustered around another sub-idea:

> Sometimes they nest in holes up in trees that are twice as high as a flagpole. Just think, the baby ducklings must jump to the ground the day they hatch. Usually they don't get hurt, though, because they're light, like little puffs of cotton. The mother stands at the foot of the tree and calls and calls. Like little paratroopers, the ducklings peek out of the hole, then jump quickly, one right after the other, to join their mother, who must hurry them to the pond where they're safe.

Thus, one of the main functions of *supporting details* is to give some dimension to a passage. Otherwise, it would be a rather uninteresting, skimpy statement of one main idea together with its bare-boned sub-ideas. The examples, descriptions, explanations and so forth are what give life to the passage.

Conclusion   As a reader moves through a passage, understanding the main idea, the sub-ideas and supporting details, it is only natural to anticipate a conclusion to the author's story. Such anticipation is part of the sport of reading. Frequently, though, the author provides the reader with a conclusion. In such an event, the joy of reading lies in the fact that the reader was able to anticipate accurately the conclusion. In the event that a conclusion is not stated, the perceptive reader will be able to seize the implied conclusion.

In the excerpts just read about the wood duck, the conclusion is in the form of having the reader visualize the pleasure of having a wood duck to observe. The concluding sentence is this:

> If you're lucky, though, and if your (duck) house is in place before the ice melts, you will have a wood duck family in the summer.

In another passage entitled "From Pond to Prairie," the author has this conclusion:

> Finally, there is no longer much open water. The pond has disappeared. Depending on the kinds of plants that have filled it, the pond may be called a bog or a marsh. As changes continue for many more years, the bog may become a forest.

The reader who reads with speed and comprehension is the reader who, like a detective, follows the maze of ideas and details and descriptions, but who is always thinking, "Where is the author leading me? What's the final point? What's the conclusion?" And, of course, like a detective, the reader must continually anticipate a conclusion, always correcting or reinforcing anticipations after taking in more and more of the story or selection.

Clarifying Devices Just as the name implies, the author uses everything possible to make the context clear and interesting. In a sense, the much-mentioned *topic sentence* may be thought of as a clarifying device. By placing it at the very beginning of a passage, the author provides the reader with an immediate point of focus, as well as a definite statement from which the reader can anticipate what is to come.

But usually, by clarifying devices, we mean the author's use of literary devices, such as transitional words and phrases which keep the ideas, sub-ideas and details in proper relationship.

To make ideas as well as details clear and interesting in themselves, authors frequently use additional literary devices such as the *metaphor*, an example of which follows: But best of all they like to eat spiders — *that's ice cream to them.*

Another literary device which authors frequently use is the *simile: Like little paratroopers*, the ducklings peek out of the hole, then jump quickly, one right after the other. The simile about the paratroopers provides the reader with familiar material that helps in visualizing the scene more graphically and vividly.

In addition to transitional words and phrases, metaphors and similes, there are many other types of *clarifying devices*. Another cluster of clarifying devices is the organizational patterns. One such pattern is the chronological organization in which the events unfold in the order of time; that is, one thing happens first, and then another, and another, and so forth.

The time pattern may give structure and control to an incident that takes place in a span of five minutes or to an historical era which may span hundreds of years. Or, used in another way, the time pattern may be the vehicle used to show the sequence of activities of an animal from birth to death or even to delineate the sequence of events in a transition.

By knowing some of these clarifying devices, you will be able to recognize them in the passages that you read, and, by recognizing them, you will be able to read with greater comprehension and with greater speed.

Vocabulary in Context

Of course, a reader who doesn't understand some of the words and terms in a passage runs the risk of misconstruing the author's ideas. It should be obvious that a reader should pause to look up in a dictionary any unfamiliar words and terms.

However, what is not so obvious is that many readers who may understand the general meaning of a word don't stop to look up such a word to ascertain its *precise* meaning.

A reader who imposes upon a generally understood word a rather general understanding, may end up with a blurred picture of the idea. Whereas, imposing a precise and full meaning upon a word immensely enhances the reader's chances of emerging with a precise and full picture of the author's ideas.

For example, in the following excerpt are two common words that most people feel they already know. Consequently, they don't see any reason for any dictionary work. Nevertheless, few people know them with the precision the words deserve.

> Depending on the kinds of plants that have filled it, the pond may be called a *bog* or a *marsh*.

Do you know the difference between a bog and a marsh? Is there a difference? If so, what is it? Would your mental picture be different if you knew?

Looking up words that you think you already know might be far more rewarding than simply seeking to add more totally unknown words to your vocabulary. In other words, strive for a smaller but precise vocabulary, rather than for a broader but slightly blurred vocabulary.

Looking up words you feel you already know will probably take more discipline than looking up unknown words. Here are some words that are likely to be unknown; so, turning to the dictionary is almost a reflex action:

> Nothing could appear more *benign* than a field aglow with daisies, goldenrod and Queen Anne's lace.

> *Sphinxlike*, it crouches among the flowers until the desired insect wanders within reach.

Thus, the dictionary is the stock market where we can exchange fuzzy meanings and soft meanings for precise meanings and where we can acquire new meaning for unknown words — and all this at no cost other than a flip of the finger.

Answering the Main Idea Question

Being able to discover the main idea of everything you read is one of the most valuable skills you can develop. The main idea questions in this book are specially designed for this development. The questions are not the ordinary multiple-choice questions; instead, each main idea question consists of four statements. Two of the statements refer to only parts of the passage. One statement states a *detail*. The aim for including a detail as an option is to provide practice in recognizing details, and not mistaking them for main ideas. The other statement is *too narrow* — it reveals more than the detail statement; nevertheless, it's too specific to be the major point of the passage.

The last two statements deal with the entire passage. One statement is *too broad*; therefore, it is too general and too vague to be an acceptable main idea statement. The remaining statement is the *main idea*. It tells *who* or *what* the subject of the passage is. In addition, the main idea statement answers the question *does what?* or *is what?*

After reading the sample passage below, follow the instructions in the box. The answer to each part of the main idea question has been filled in for you, as well as the score for each answer.

Sample

The steel trap's jaws had caught the coyote midway across the foot. The pain must have been awful. Yet the coyote never stopped trying to tear loose. It had dug a circle about six inches (about 15.2 centimeters) deep, stretching the full length of the steel chain.

Two young boys out hiking saw this trapped coyote. They hurried to a nearby ranch. The ranch owner heard them out and came to help.

They held the coyote's neck down firmly with hoe handles. Then they opened the trap's jaws. The coyote slipped free. But the animal stayed there, just looking at its helpers. Perhaps it was wondering what makes some people demons and others saints.

The animal had to be gently nudged before it would leave. At last, it hobbled off a short distance. Then it turned, pausing to look again at the good people who had spared its life.

	Answer	Score
Mark the main idea	M	10
Mark the statement that is a detail	D	5
Mark the statement that is too narrow	N	5
Mark the statement that is too broad	B	5

a. Two young boys helped to free a trapped coyote.
   [This statement is a summary that gathers all the essential points to give an accurate picture of the main idea in a brief way: (a) two young boys, (b) a trapped coyote, and (c) freeing it.]

b. Kind hearts set free a doomed coyote.
   [This statement is too general. It doesn't state *who* set the coyote free or *why* it was doomed.]

c. Hoe handles were used to hold the coyote down.
   [This is only one of many details mentioned in the passage. It has little to do with the passage as a whole.]

d. A steel trap was opened to set a coyote free.
   [Opening the trap is *part* of the main idea. But any main idea statement must give the chief actors credit. It must include the two boys who were responsible for freeing the coyote.]

Getting the Most Out of This Book

The following steps might be called "tricks of the trade" by readers, while your teachers might call them "rules for learning." It doesn't matter what they are called, though; what does matter is that they work.

Think About the Title

An internationally famous linguist informed me of a "trick" to use every time I read: "The first thing to do is to read the title and spend a few moments thinking about it."

Writers take considerable time inventing intriguing titles. They attempt to pack them with meaning. Consequently, it is common sense for you to spend a few seconds trying to discover some meaning. These initial moments of thought will enable you to increase your understanding of the passage before you even read it.

Thinking about the title can assist comprehension in another way, also. It helps you concentrate on a passage before you actually begin reading. Thinking about the title fills your head so full of thoughts about the passage that there's simply no room for anything else to enter to disrupt concentration.

The Dot System

Here is a step that will speed up your reading and develop comprehension at the same time.

After spending a few moments considering the title, *quickly* read through the passage. Then, without looking back, answer the six questions by placing a dot in the appropriate box beside each answer of your choice. The dots will serve as your "unofficial" answers. For the main idea question (question six), place your dot in the box alongside the statement that you consider the main idea.

The dot system improves your reading comprehension by making you work harder on an initial, *fast* reading. The practice you acquire by trying to understand and retain ideas makes you a stronger reader.

The Check-Mark System

After you have answered all of the questions using a dot, read the passage again, *carefully*, but this time, indicate your final answer to each question using a check mark (✓). For each question, place a check mark in the appropriate box next to the answer of your choice. The answers with the check marks are the "official" ones that will be counted toward your score.

To answer the main idea questions, follow the special instructions given on each question page. Use a capital letter to indicate your final answer to each option in the main idea question.

The Diagnostic Chart

Now transfer your final answers to the Diagnostic Chart on page 102. Use the column of boxes under number *1* for the answers to the first passage. Use the column of boxes under number *2* for the answers to the second passage, and so on.

Write the letter of your answer in the *upper* portion of each block.

Correct your answers using the Answer Key on page 100. When scoring your answers, do *not* use an *x* for *incorrect* or a *c* for *correct*. Instead, follow this procedure: if your answer is correct, make no mark in the lower portion of the answer block. If your answer is *in*correct, however, write the letter of the correct answer in the *lower* portion of the block.

Properly used, therefore, the answer column for the individual passages will indicate not only your incorrect answers, but also the correct answers.

Your Total Comprehension Score

Return to the passage you have just finished reading. If you answered a question incorrectly, underline the correct response on the question page. Then write your score for each question in the circles provided. Finally, add the scores to determine your Total Comprehension Score.

Graphing Your Progress

After you have computed your Total Comprehension Score, turn to the Progress Graph on page 103. Transfer your score to the box under the number for each passage. Then put an *x* along the line above the box to indicate your Total Comprehension Score. Connect the *x*'s as you read through the book; plot a line showing your comprehension development.

Taking Corrective Action

Your incorrect answers will provide you with a valuable opportunity for self-teaching if you take a moment to consider your mistakes.

Return to the original question and read the correct answer (the one you previously underlined) several times. With the correct answer in mind, go back to the passage itself and read to understand why the approved answer is better. Try to discover where you made your mistake. Try to determine why you chose an incorrect answer.

The Steps in a Nutshell

Here's a quick review of the steps to follow in order to get the most out of each *Essential Skills* book. Be sure you have carefully read and understood all the information in the "To the Student" section (pages 11 to 22) before you begin.

1. **Think About the Title of the Passsage.** Try to get all the meaning the writer put into it.
2. **Read the Passage Quickly.**
3. **Answer the Questions, Using the Dot System.** Use dots to indicate your unofficial answers. Don't look back at the passage.
4. **Read the Passage Again — Carefully.**
5. **Make Your Final Answers.** Place a check mark (✓) in the box to indicate your final answer. Use capital letters for each part of the main idea question.
6. **Transfer Your Answers to the Diagnostic Chart.** Record your final answers in the upper blocks of the chart on page 102.
7. **Correct Your Answers.** Use the Answer Key on pages 100 and 101. If an answer is incorrect, (a) write the correct answer in the lower block, underneath your wrong answer; and (b) go back to the original question and underline the correct answer.
8. **Calculate Your Total Comprehension Score.** Calculate your Total Comprehension Score by adding up the points you earned for each question.
9. **Graph Your Progress.** Record and plot your scores on the graph on page 103.
10. **Take Corrective Action.** Learn from your incorrect answers by reading the passage again and trying to determine the reason you were wrong.

Passages and Questions

Titles of Passages

1. Wonders of the Wild: The Cassowary 24
2. Bite 'em Back 27
3. The Incredible Mystery of Migration 30
4. The Roadrunner 33
5. Vanished but Not Forgotten 36
6. Why I Hunt 39
7. More Giants 42
8. The Red Squirrel 45
9. The Raccoon 48
10. The Spring Peeper 51
11. Under and Above Ground 54
12. Leave Them Alone! 57
13. Moving Rocks for Locks 60
14. Salt Water Bait Too 63
15. Snow As an Insulator 66
16. That Butterfly Is Really a Clam! 69
17. Hippie of the Feathered World 72
18. The Most Ferocious Animal in the Woods 75
19. The Buffalo Hunters 78
20. Foxy Family 81
21. The Red Fox As a Hunter 84
22. Pop-Out and Fall-Away Seeds 87
23. Temporary Tines 90
24. Christmas Trees 93
25. The Bird That Survived 96

1. Wonders of the Wild: The Cassowary

The cassowary (KASS oh wary) crashed through the New Guinea jungle, determined to kill the human fleeing ahead of her. She traveled at an unbelievable speed — averaging thirty miles (about 48.3 kilometers) an hour! The bony helmet on her forehead acted as a battering ram smashing aside the undergrowth; her coarse, hairlike feathers protected her from the brambles and branches.

The human, a New Guinean, had wandered unintentionally into her nesting area and was terrified. The human ran at maximum speed, aware of being chased by one of the most dangerous animals on the island. Many other islanders had been killed by cassowaries — these birds are about five feet (about 1.5 meters) tall and weigh over 100 pounds (about 45.4 kilograms)! They first run down their victims, then leap at them feet first, lashing out with their powerful claws. The inner claw, a sharply pointed, five-inch-long (about 12.7-centimeter-long) nail, is a deadly weapon.

The islander spotted a tree and clambered up just as the cassowary burst through the <u>undergrowth</u>. She smashed into the tree, battering it with her head and slashing it with her claws. But because she could not fly, her prey was safe. The cassowary eventually forgot the chase and went crashing back through the jungle toward her nest. The islander ran home safely.

The cassowary's mate remained on the nest, a slightly raised platform of leaves on the jungle floor. He was smaller than the female and, except at mating and breeding seasons, avoided her. Five peagreen eggs lay in the nest; each were six inches (about 15.2 centimeters) long and weighed more than one pound (about .45 kilograms). It was the male cassowary's responsibility to incubate them. After the female cassowary had contributed the eggs, she had wandered away, leaving her mate to occupy the nest for lengthy periods of time. When he became hungry, he dashed into the jungle and stripped berries from bushes or consumed lizards and small birds. Then he lumbered back to the nest and its eggs. Meanwhile, the female cassowary took her time, hunting or sleeping away the tropical days. She stayed near the nest to guard it only until the eggs hatched, seven weeks after being laid.

The chicks were tiny, brown-and-white striped birds and were completely helpless. Both parents devoted themselves to them until they were able to leave the nest and get along by themselves. If they escaped the jungle's dangers, they too would become powerful and bad-tempered like their parents.

The cassowary has nothing that attracts people: its feathers are not wanted, its flesh is not nutritious to eat, and the remote jungle it inhabits is not good for farming or for constructing cities. So, for the time being, it will remain unmolested and free to go crashing through the jungle — another of the countless wonders of the wild.

?

		Possible Score	Your Score

1. The cassowary is a

    ☐ a. native.
    ☐ b. snake.
    ☐ c. bird.
    ☐ d. lizard.

    (15)   ◯

2. How fast can a cassowary move?

    ☐ a. A few feet (about 1 meter) in one hour
    ☐ b. 30 miles (about 48.3 kilometers) an hour
    ☐ c. 4 or 5 feet (about 1.2–1.5 meters) in a day
    ☐ d. 60 or 70 miles (about 96.6–112.7 kilometers) an hour

    (15)   ◯

3. After reading this passage, we can see that cassowaries are

    ☐ a. very friendly.
    ☐ b. quite shy.
    ☐ c. somewhat weak.
    ☐ d. strong and bad-tempered.

    (15)   ◯

4. The native in this passage must have felt

    ☐ a. sorry for the cassowary.
    ☐ b. guilty.
    ☐ c. terrified.
    ☐ d. happy about finding the cassowary.

    (15)   ◯

5. The underguard of a jungle refers to its

    ☐ a. plants.
    ☐ b. animals.
    ☐ c. rocky area.
    ☐ d. lakes.

    (15)   ◯

6. Main Idea

	Answer	Score
Mark the main idea	M	10
Mark the statement that is a detail	D	5
Mark the statement that is too narrow	N	5
Mark the statement that is too broad	B	5

a. Cassowaries can kill a human with their dangerous claws.

b. There are birds quite different from the ones in your backyard.

c. The cassowary is a large, dangerous and fierce New Guinea bird.

d. The flightless cassowary can run at 30 miles (about 48.3 kilometers) per hour.

Total Comprehension Score
(Add your scores and enter the total on the graph on page 103.)

Categories of Comprehension Questions

No. 1: Subject Matter	No. 4: Clarifying Devices
No. 2: Supporting Details	No. 5: Vocabulary in Context
No. 3: Conclusion	No. 6: Main Idea

2. Bite 'em Back

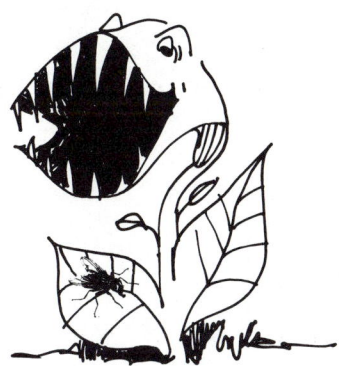

Animals have been dining on plants since life on earth began, but there are a few plants — four families of them, in fact — that turn the tables and bite back at the animal world: the sundew, the pitcher plant, the Venus's-flytrap and the bladderwort.

All have specialized leaves that act as baited traps. When insects spring these traps, their meaty juices are digested by specialized plant cells, and the plants get a meal of nitrogen to make up for lack of that essential element in the coastal, flatland bogs where they live.

There are many species of sundews scattered over the world. Typically, they have small, paddle-shaped leaves. The upper surfaces of the leaves support many tentacles which are tipped with tiny balls of mucilage. Insects, attracted by this glistening sap, alight and become trapped — and digested.

The Venus's-flytrap catches insects in a more dramatic fashion. Mouths of the traps have trigger hairs on the inside. If two or more of the hairs are touched, the spiny leaves snap shut and form a tight purse around the prey. The digestive process takes about ten days, after which the lobes reopen. Restricted to the coastal plain of the Carolinas, the Venus's-flytrap has suffered a great reduction in number in the last few years from collectors, drainage and encroaching "progress."

Both the flowers and the leaves of the pitcher plants are unusually attractive. The leaves of the different species vary a great deal and have been termed "astonishing culminations of anatomical evolution." They have one thing in common — a hollow, tubular reservoir in the leaf, often lined with downward-pointing hairs leading to a small amount of fluid at the end of the cavity. The hairs serve as a one-way street for the ants, mites and other insects which find their way into the passage, and their fate is to drown in the super-wet digestive fluid at the end of the road.

Some carnivorous plants are baited with sweet-smelling nectar and some with odors like rotting meat. The cobra-lily's semitransparent dome serves as a <u>visual</u> <u>lure</u>, and this "studio skylight" also keeps the interior of the plant warm and "cozy."

How could any insect resist?

_____ **?** _____

	Possible Score	Your Score

1. The author of this passage is discussing certain kinds of

   ☐ a. insects.
   ☐ b. animals.
   ☐ c. plants.
   ☐ d. flatland bogs.

   (15)   ◯

2. Where does the Venus's-flytrap live?

   ☐ a. The river banks of the Mississippi River
   ☐ b. The coastal plains of the Carolinas
   ☐ c. The mountain areas of New England
   ☐ d. The deserts of North America

   (15)   ◯

3. It seems that soil from swamp areas is low in

   ☐ a. oxygen.
   ☐ b. nitrogen.
   ☐ c. hydrogen.
   ☐ d. phosphates.

   (15)   ◯

4. The Venus's-flytrap catches insects in a "dramatic fashion." This means the Venus's-flytrap is

   ☐ a. boring.
   ☐ b. humorous.
   ☐ c. exciting.
   ☐ d. apathetic.

   (15)   ◯

5. A <u>visual</u> lure has to be

   ☐ a. heard.
   ☐ b. tasted.
   ☐ c. touched.
   ☐ d. seen.

   (15)   ◯

6. Main Idea

	Answer	Score
Mark the main idea	M	10
Mark the statement that is a detail	D	5
Mark the statement that is too narrow	N	5
Mark the statement that is too broad	B	5

a. Sundews have small, paddle-shaped leaves.

b. A few plants have turned the tables on insects.

c. Venus's fly-traps digest an insect in 10 days.

d. Some plants trap and digest insects.

Total Comprehension Score
(Add your scores and enter the
total on the graph on page 103.)

Categories of Comprehension Questions

No. 1: Subject Matter   No. 4: Clarifying Devices

No. 2: Supporting Details   No. 5: Vocabulary in Context

No. 3: Conclusion   No. 6: Main Idea

3. The Incredible Mystery of Migration

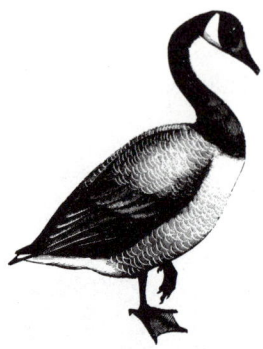

The old Canadian goose was feeling restless and irritable. The sun cut a lower arc across the sky each day, far south of the nesting grounds, and each day the old bird had a greater feeling of urgency, of agitation.

Finally, the feeling became too strong to bear. Late one afternoon, after <u>gorging</u> itself on everything it could find, it could no longer stand the feeling and, spreading its mighty wings, it turned into the wind and heaved itself into the air. As if on signal, scores of others in the flock followed, forming themselves into a great V that spread across the sky.

The old goose wheeled south as the low sun set, and its throbbing wings carried it into the black night.

It led the flock down the belly of the continent, stopping to feed and rest or wait out the weather, but always returning to the invisible path that millions of its ancestors had cruised before. There were few landmarks on the dark surface of the earth to guide it, and it seems likely that those it could see stirred no memories. Sometimes the flock rested, but always there was the drive to beat south, south.

It took several days to travel the invisible route, but the flock would not be stopped. At last the old goose, as though heading straight into the landing pattern of an airport, brought them safely to the Louisiana marshes that had served as wintering quarters for thousands of its ancestors.

Months later, as the sun moved north across the blue dome of the heavens, it would again feel the strange restlessness, the compulsion to take to the sky and wheel northward. And again it would soar without error back to the same small area of land, lost in the vast wilderness of Canada, that had served as the nesting grounds of hundreds of generations before it.

How does it do it? How can a bird perform this remarkable act of navigation twice each year? The old goose is but one of millions of birds and animals that leave their homes and set out on journeys without a remembered goal and along routes that many of them have never seen before.

_____ **?** _____

	Possible Score	Your Score

1. To show migration, the passage discusses the

   ☐ a. Canadian goose.
   ☐ b. swallow.
   ☐ c. stork.
   ☐ d. butterfly.   (15)   ◯

2. Where did this flock land?

   ☐ a. Texas
   ☐ b. Florida
   ☐ c. Nova Scotia
   ☐ d. Louisiana   (15)   ◯

3. It can be seen that the urge to migrate is probably

   ☐ a. learned.
   ☐ b. acquired.
   ☐ c. in-born.
   ☐ d. dying out.   (15)   ◯

4. At what time of day would you see a "low sun"?

   ☐ a. Midmorning
   ☐ b. Noontime
   ☐ c. Afternoon
   ☐ d. Sunset   (15)   ◯

5. As used in this passage, gorging means

   ☐ a. eating.
   ☐ b. flying.
   ☐ c. mating.
   ☐ d. preening.   (15)   ◯

6. Main Idea

	Answer	Score
Mark the main idea	M	10
Mark the statement that is a detail	D	5
Mark the statement that is too narrow	N	5
Mark the statement that is too broad	B	5

a. Some birds feel a mysterious urge to travel twice a year.

b. Birds migrate by instinct and without errors twice a year.

c. Canadian geese fly to the Louisiana marshes for winter.

d. Canadian geese fly in a great V formation in the sky.

Total Comprehension Score
(Add your scores and enter the total on the graph on page 103.)

Categories of Comprehension Questions

No. 1: Subject Matter	No. 4: Clarifying Devices
No. 2: Supporting Details	No. 5: Vocabulary in Context
No. 3: Conclusion	No. 6: Main Idea

4. The Roadrunner

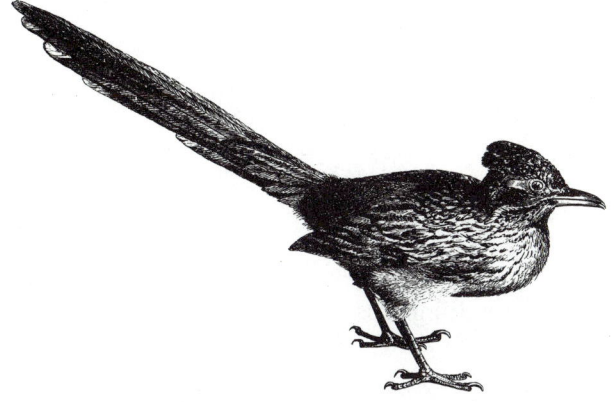

Many birds avoid the driest desert, but the roadrunner stays in it through all seasons and it seems actually to prefer the regions which are hottest and driest. You will find it nesting among the murderous spines of the cholla — wickedest of all the cacti — and searching the area for lizards and snakes which are its preferred food and with which it feeds its young.

It can fly well enough to reach the lower limbs of the trees if it has to, but it prefers to trust its long legs both to catch its prey and to keep out of trouble. The sounds which it makes are neither birdlike nor very much like anything else. It can, on occasion, make a strange noise that is a sort of raucous coo, but it usually prefers a rapid clashing of its bill, making a surprisingly loud noise not to be forgotten.

In hard seasons it will eat the larger insects, leaping to take in flight a dragonfly or other creatures substantial enough to be worth the trouble. But its favorite food is reptilian. It catches lizards after chasing them wildly from bush to bush, and it is said that they cannot escape from it as they do from other predators by shedding their tails. The roadrunner knows that trick and swallows the body first, leaving the wiggling tail for later.

Snakes — including rattlers — however, seem to be what it likes best, and there is no odder sight than a roadrunner in the hours-long process of disposing of an eighteen-inch (about 45.7-centimeter) snake. It goes about its other business with the unswallowed portion dangling from its mouth, and it gradually disappears as the other end is digested.

All these peculiarities and adaptations are things learned rather recently. The roadrunner is not a creature that happened to have certain characteristics which fitted it for desert life. When it gradually moved into regions that were more and more arid, it must have been a part of the cuckoo bird family. Other cuckoos fly, sing and live mostly on insects. Now it is a cuckoo bird only to those who can interpret the evidence hidden in its anatomy. To the rest of us, it is a desert bird, as much a part of the desert as the cholla in which it nests.

?

	Possible Score	Your Score

1. The roadrunner is

   ☐ a. a bird.
   ☐ b. a snake.
   ☐ c. a rodent.
   ☐ d. a lizard.

   15

2. The favorite food of the roadrunner is

   ☐ a. the cholla.
   ☐ b. reptiles.
   ☐ c. algae.
   ☐ d. seeds.

   15

3. It appears that the roadrunner is related to

   ☐ a. the dragonfly.
   ☐ b. the toad.
   ☐ c. the Gila woodpecker.
   ☐ d. the cuckoo.

   15

4. The author feels that the roadrunner is

   ☐ a. endangered.
   ☐ b. peculiar.
   ☐ c. elegant.
   ☐ d. delicate.

   15

5. The <u>limbs</u> of a tree are its

   ☐ a. leaves.
   ☐ b. seeds.
   ☐ c. roots.
   ☐ d. branches.

   15

6. Main Idea

	Answer	Score
Mark the main idea	M	(10)
Mark the statement that is a detail	D	(5)
Mark the statement that is too narrow	N	(5)
Mark the statement that is too broad	B	(5)

a. The roadrunner is well adapted to desert life.

b. Roadrunners seem to prefer the desert.

c. Roadrunners nest in cacti just as other birds nest in trees.

d. The favorite foods of roadrunners are lizards and snakes.

Total Comprehension Score
(Add your scores and enter the total on the graph on page 103.)

Categories of Comprehension Questions

No. 1: Subject Matter	No. 4: Clarifying Devices
No. 2: Supporting Details	No. 5: Vocabulary in Context
No. 3: Conclusion	No. 6: Main Idea

5. Vanished but Not Forgotten

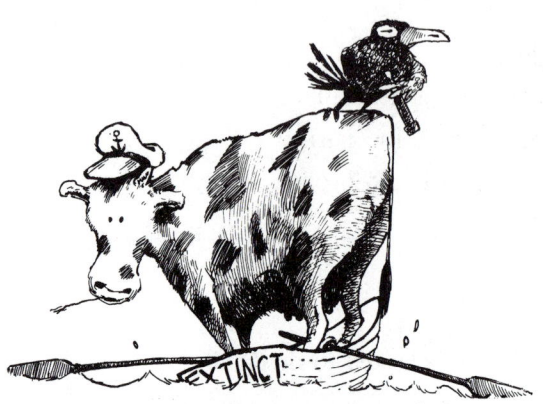

It is not always quite so easy to pinpoint the <u>extermination</u> of a species. For example, the full reason behind the extinction of the beautiful black-and-white Labrador duck has never been established.

This duck migrated down the United States east coast in large numbers each fall, and it never failed to run into lethal gunners who would down the pretty bird for its plumage or meat. Almost before anyone realized it, the birds had become extremely rare and what few remained were probably destroyed by Canadian Indians who raided what nests and eggs they could find.

The Labrador duck became a tragic statistic when, on December 12, 1875, a duck hunter on Long Island shot and killed a large male bird. It was the last Labrador duck.

One of our most deplorable extinctions came about in 1844 when the last of those magnificent sea birds, the great auks, were slain. Rather penguinlike in appearance, they nested on the rocky islands and coasts of the North Atlantic, from Iceland to Greenland, Labrador and Newfoundland. Each autumn they migrated down our east coast, often as far as 3,000 miles (about 4,828 kilometers) from where they started, and each spring they would swim back to their isolated rocks to lay a single egg per mated pair.

Isolated though these rocks were, they weren't distant enough to protect the auks from humans. The auk's thick plumage, almost like heavy fur, was much in demand as down for bedding. The huge eggs were delicious and were much sought after by sailors. The flesh was a cheap, easy source of fresh meat, and even the body oils were put to use.

The great auks would stand helplessly at their rocky island nesting sites, watching the hunters approach. Hundreds, even thousands of them would fall to the clubs of people who herded them into dense clusters to begin their grisly work. It was on June 3, 1844, on the island of Eldey, off Iceland's southwestern coast, that a nesting pair of great auks were slain by Jon Brandsson and Sigourour Isleffson. Their single egg was smashed by Ketil Ketilsson, and the great auk was forever lost to the world.

_____ ? _____

	Possible Score	Your Score

1. This passage focuses on

   ☐ a. the wood duck and the penguin.
   ☐ b. the Labrador duck and the great auks.
   ☐ c. Canadian geese and the albatross.
   ☐ d. herons and the Arctic tern.

   (15) ◯

2. Canadian Indians raided the nests of

   ☐ a. the Labrador duck.
   ☐ b. the great auks.
   ☐ c. Canadian geese.
   ☐ d. the wood duck.

   (15) ◯

3. This passage suggests that the foremost cause of extinction is

   ☐ a. overhunting.
   ☐ b. disease.
   ☐ c. climatic changes.
   ☐ d. low birth rate.

   (15) ◯

4. Which of the following describes the overall tone of this passage?

   ☐ a. Indifferent
   ☐ b. Sarcastic
   ☐ c. Humorous
   ☐ d. Tragic

   (15) ◯

5. Another word for <u>extermination</u> is

   ☐ a. expansion.
   ☐ b. resolution.
   ☐ c. destruction.
   ☐ d. subjection.

   (15) ◯

6. Main Idea

	Answer	Score
Mark the main idea	M	10
Mark the statement that is a detail	D	5
Mark the statement that is too narrow	N	5
Mark the statement that is too broad	B	5

a. The Labrador duck had beautiful black and white feathers.

b. Hunting can contribute to wildlife extinction.

c. Auks and Labrador ducks are extinct because of hunting.

d. The great auks were killed for their feathers and meat.

Total Comprehension Score
(Add your scores and enter the total on the graph on page 103.)

Categories of Comprehension Questions

No. 1: Subject Matter	No. 4: Clarifying Devices
No. 2: Supporting Details	No. 5: Vocabulary in Context
No. 3: Conclusion	No. 6: Main Idea

6. Why I Hunt

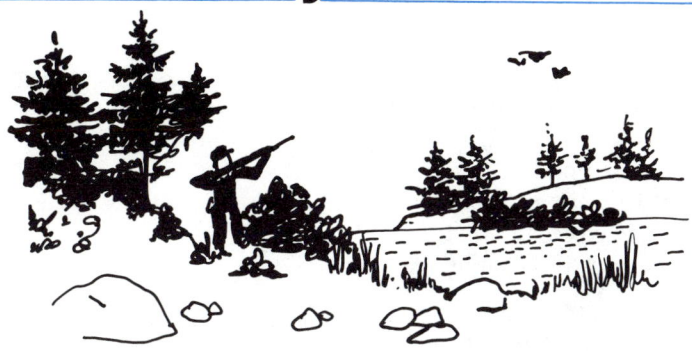

No one could be more willing to recommend hunting as a wholesome form of outdoor recreation than I. For one thing, I believe hunting has many values for those who participate in it. I like to think of it as being more than just a sport. It's a form of recreation which brings many physical, mental and even spiritual benefits to the individual.

The person in the blind who is crouched down watching the on-coming flock of geese isn't worrying about income tax. The child whose "big thrill" is a jaunt in the woods with a gun and dog doesn't come before the juvenile court judge. Hunters don't suffer from sleepless nights (unless it's the night before the opening day) and very, very few develop ulcers.

Hunting does other things for people, too. Hunters learn early that sportsmanship and good field etiquette are essential. They learn to respect and love the wild animals they pursue. They discover the pleasures of the things they see, hear and smell as they walk through field and forest or paddle through the duck marsh. Many develop a reverence for all nature and everywhere see the handiwork of a higher power in the out-of-doors.

It's not too hard to defend hunting, as well as the hunter. Those who think of guns and bullets as inhumane don't understand the ways of nature very well. Everything in the wild could be classified as inhumane and cruel. The life expectancy of the smaller birds and mammals is shockingly short. For the common cottontail rabbit, favorite quarry of the gunner, it's only a matter of a few weeks. Only a small percentage ever see their first birthday, with or without hunting.

Nature's creatures die by the talon and fang, from diseases, parasites and from all kinds of accidents. Dying by the hunter's gun is quicker and more merciful than starvation and probably less cruel than being torn apart by a hawk, owl or fox.

The hunter only takes some of those animals which are doomed anyway, usually a very small part. And I believe that using these surpluses for recreation and for food makes just as much sense as raising cattle, hogs and sheep to slaughter. And I doubt whether shooting a deer or a pheasant is any more cruel or inhumane than shooting a steer and cutting out its steaks for the very people who criticize the sport. Perhaps we should adopt the rule that no one should condemn hunting unless they are strict vegetarians.

_____ **?** _____

		Possible Score	Your Score

1. What would be another good title for this passage?

   ☐ a. Hunting for Food
   ☐ b. Natural Enemies of Humans
   ☐ c. Hunting Farms Are Great
   ☐ d. The Pleasures of Hunting   (15)   ◯

2. The hunter in this passage uses

   ☐ a. guns and bullets.
   ☐ b. a bow and arrows.
   ☐ c. a camera.
   ☐ d. snare traps.   (15)   ◯

3. The writer suggests that most cottontail rabbits

   ☐ a. live in well-hidden burrows.
   ☐ b. die before they are a year old.
   ☐ c. are not afraid of people.
   ☐ d. can make good pets.   (15)   ◯

4. The author of this passage

   ☐ a. believes in hunting farms.
   ☐ b. clearly enjoys hunting.
   ☐ c. thinks hunting is inhumane.
   ☐ d. finds hunting very boring.   (15)   ◯

5. A child might enjoy a <u>jaunt</u> in the woods. As used in this passage, a *jaunt* is a

   ☐ a. fishing spot.
   ☐ b. blind.
   ☐ c. campsite.
   ☐ d. short walk.   (15)   ◯

6. Main Idea

	Answer	Score
Mark the main idea	M	10
Mark the statement that is a detail	D	5
Mark the statement that is too narrow	N	5
Mark the statement that is too broad	B	5

a. Hunting is a pleasurable, worthwhile sport.

b. Hunters learn to respect nature.

c. Many people have the wrong idea about hunting.

d. Most wild animals have very short life spans.

Total Comprehension Score
(Add your scores and enter the
total on the graph on page 103.)

Categories of Comprehension Questions

No. 1: Subject Matter	No. 4: Clarifying Devices
No. 2: Supporting Details	No. 5: Vocabulary in Context
No. 3: Conclusion	No. 6: Main Idea

7. More Giants

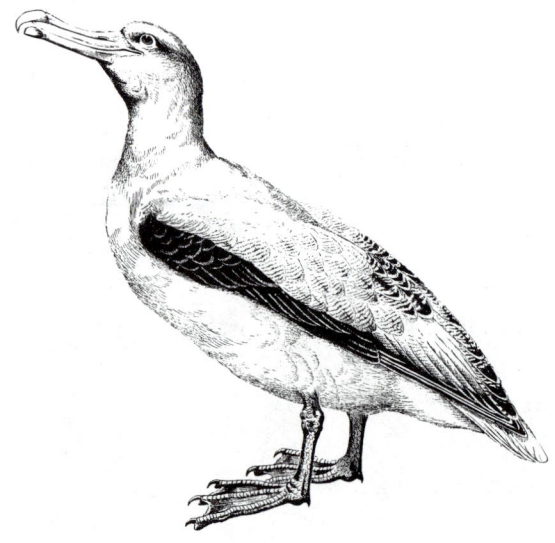

Of the flying birds, the South African gom-paauw (kori bustard) tips the scale as the heaviest. Some specimens weigh more than forty pounds (about 18.1 kilograms), which is a lot of weight to flap into the air. The bird with the largest wingspan, however, is the wandering albatross, that remarkable soarer of the southern seas which has inspired many a fable and poem. Its wingspan is a record-breaker: up to twelve feet (about 3.7 meters) or more, but it has the unique ability to drink sea water and separate out the salt.

A true horror is the salt-water crocodile of Southeast Asia, largest of all the reptiles. One recorded specimen was thirty-three feet (about 10.1 meters) long and weighed more than three tons (about 2.7 tonnes). This creature isn't kidding, either; strictly carnivorous, it lives in the tidal waters and will eat any available meat, including unwary humans.

But *Homo sapiens*, in all their glory, have made size unimportant. Because of its enormity, an elephant once could rule its section of the earth without fear. Now a pellet no larger than a human thumb can bring it thundering to the ground. The largest creature on this planet once roamed the icy seas in great numbers. Now a child's finger on the trigger of a harpoon gun can make those seas run scarlet with the blood of the earth's greatest creature, the blue whale.

Humans stand supreme — *the* giants of the earth — except for their greatest enemies, viruses and bacteria, so small that we can see them only with the most powerful microscopes. Perhaps not the giants, but the midgets, may someday inherit the earth the giants once trod.

_____ **?** _____

	Possible Score	Your Score

1. What would be another good title for this passage?

   ☐ a. Who's Kidding Who?
   ☐ b. That's the Size of It!
   ☐ c. Horrors of the Salt Water
   ☐ d. It's H-E-A-V-Y

   (15)   ◯

2. The salt-water crocodile of Southeast Asia can weigh more than

   ☐ a. 3 tons (about 2.7 tonnes).
   ☐ b. the blue whale.
   ☐ c. 30 tons (about 27 tonnes).
   ☐ d. the African elephant.

   (15)   ◯

3. The largest animal on this earth is a

   ☐ a. bird.
   ☐ b. sea creature.
   ☐ c. land animal.
   ☐ d. tree dweller.

   (15)   ◯

4. The word "pellet" refers to a

   ☐ a. marble.
   ☐ b. ball of food.
   ☐ c. small pill.
   ☐ d. bullet.

   (15)   ◯

5. <u>Scarlet</u> is a shade of

   ☐ a. blue.
   ☐ b. red.
   ☐ c. yellow.
   ☐ d. orange.

   (15)   ◯

6. Main Idea

	Answer	Score
Mark the main idea	M	10
Mark the statement that is a detail	D	5
Mark the statement that is too narrow	N	5
Mark the statement that is too broad	B	5

a. Though not the largest, humans are the most powerful creatures.

b. 40 pounds (about 18.1 kilograms) is a lot of weight for a bird to lift.

c. The biggest animals are not the most successful.

d. The largest whale can be killed by one human with a harpoon.

Total Comprehension Score
(Add your scores and enter the total on the graph on page 103.)

Categories of Comprehension Questions

No. 1: Subject Matter	No. 4: Clarifying Devices
No. 2: Supporting Details	No. 5: Vocabulary in Context
No. 3: Conclusion	No. 6: Main Idea

8. The Red Squirrel

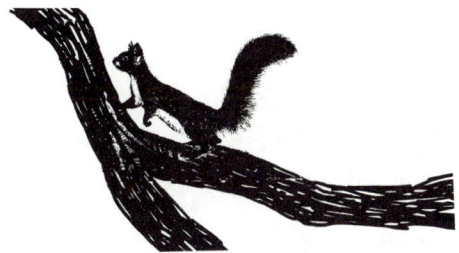

The red squirrel enters the world in late May or early June, depending upon the severity of the winter, with three or four litter-mates. It is the mother who does all the feeding and provides protective care. Snug in a carefully made nest of shredded, softened bark, covered on the outside with heavy grasses, the naked little babies grow rapidly and, in a little over a week, usually have their eyes open. In time they will become a deep golden red with a black line running along each side in summer and a whitish belly. Later in the fall, the stripes will fade, the color will darken somewhat and fuzzy tufts will spring up on the tips of the ears like misplaced earmuffs.

When the little ones venture from the nest for the first time, they are in for a rude shock. Their abode is well out on a flimsy limb, anywhere from ten to forty feet (about 3.1 to 12.2 meters) above the ground. Mom has given a lot of thought to locating the nest so that, if possible, it is out of reach of heavier predators like bobcats, weasels, pine marten and other climbing meat eaters. Her constant worry is the unavoidable flying killers of the forest who'll try for a tasty morsel of squirrel meat every chance they get.

From the day they first discover how far down that old ground is, the little half-grown babes must start learning to find food, protect themselves from a hundred seen and unseen enemies, run, climb and bathe. This last step is a very important one because the main food of the red squirrel is seeds from the cones of spruce, pine and other evergreens, and they are covered with pitch. Unless the tiny paws are cleaned meticulously every few minutes, the animal would soon be disabled by the accumulated gum.

One sure way to spot a nesting area is to look for a pile of *scales*, the inedible portions of pine cones discarded after the tiny bit of nutlike meat has been eaten from the seeds. These flutter to the ground, quickly forming a big pile because many cones must be shredded to provide a full meal for the tiny belly. Later, these scales will be the basic part of the *midden* or storehouse for food laid away for the future. The midden may be huge, or it may be fairly small — the latter indicating that there are a large number of similar storehouses close by. One big midden found by researchers measured eighteen feet (about 5.5 meters) long by five feet, six inches (about 1.7 meters) wide, and a careful tally revealed 4,609 stored cones! During the time the count was being made, a sharp, penetrating scolding was being delivered with vigor. It ceased only when the entire stock was reburied, and the intruders silently left, betting that the little one in the tree was going to come down and tally its hoard cone by cone.

?

	Possible Score	Your Score

1. This passage tells us about

    ☐ a. young red squirrels.
    ☐ b. mating habits of the red squirrel.
    ☐ c. the way squirrels fight.
    ☐ d. the male red squirrels.

    (15)

2. What does the red squirrel eat?

    ☐ a. Fish
    ☐ b. Small field rodents
    ☐ c. Insects
    ☐ d. Seeds from evergreens

    (15)

3. We can see that

    ☐ a. baby squirrels are helpless and need care.
    ☐ b. red squirrels are becoming extinct.
    ☐ c. female squirrels are aggressive.
    ☐ d. strong, sturdy branches are used to build a squirrel nest.

    (15)

4. A squirrel's "litter-mates" are its

    ☐ a. parents.
    ☐ b. enemies.
    ☐ c. brothers and sisters.
    ☐ d. middens.

    (15)

5. A good synonym for vigor is

    ☐ a. disgust.
    ☐ b. strength.
    ☐ c. anger.
    ☐ d. curiosity.

    (15)

6. Main Idea

	Answer	Score
Mark the main idea	M	10
Mark the statement that is a detail	D	5
Mark the statement that is too narrow	N	5
Mark the statement that is too broad	B	5

a. Red squirrels are born 10 to 40 feet (about 3.1 to 12.2 meters) above the ground.

b. Red squirrels store their pine cones for food in winter.

c. Red squirrels learn everything they need to survive.

d. Forest creatures must take care of themselves.

Total Comprehension Score
(Add your scores and enter the total on the graph on page 103.)

Categories of Comprehension Questions

No. 1: Subject Matter	No. 4: Clarifying Devices
No. 2: Supporting Details	No. 5: Vocabulary in Context
No. 3: Conclusion	No. 6: Main Idea

9. The Raccoon

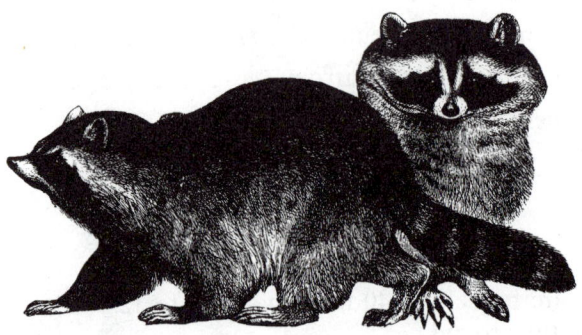

The life of a raccoon begins in a secluded den, usually in a hollow tree where the rain has rotted a hole or where a large limb has fallen off leaving an entrance. Following the gestation period of about sixty-three days, the female produces a litter of four to six young. They leave the den some ten weeks later to accompany their mother on her nightly food-hunting trip. In the fall the family separates.

At that time, the youngster is truly on its own and has acquired most of its food-gathering techniques. But not entirely, for the raccoon is everlastingly curious and leaves few stones unturned when it goes in search of food.

In the matter of menu, the raccoon displays a kinship to people. It is *omniverous*, eating nearly everything that comes along whether it be meat or vegetable. Its flesh diet is largely made up of small birds and mammals, fish, frogs, snails, mussels, crayfish, insects, and so forth. Various vegetable products are included in the diet at all times of the year.

Experiments and observations reveal that acorns are eaten very extensively during all seasons, even winter. Grapes and other fruits are eaten during the fall. Corn in the "milk" stage is especially relished.

In olden times the raccoon's worst enemies were the wolf and panther. With the removal of these two animals, the raccoon was practically without an enemy. A full-grown raccoon can put up a good fight when cornered, and many a dog has regretted an encounter with the spunky animal. Disease takes its toll, however, and raccoons are subject to the same periodic "die-offs" that plague the fox family. Young raccoons, too, may fall prey to owls and night-roving animals. No longer is the pelt in great demand as it once was, but the decade-old "Davy Crockett" trend focused attention on its worth for a brief span.

Raccoon hunting is a major sporting activity in areas of Tennessee where they are abundant. A good dog is given a hearty workout when sent in search of the scent of this black-masked eluder.

?

		Possible Score	Your Score
1.	What would be another good title for this passage? ☐ a. How the Raccoon Got Its Mask ☐ b. The Family Life of Woodland Creatures ☐ c. Raccoons and Colonial Hunters ☐ d. Let's Talk About Raccoons	15	○
2.	The gestation period for the raccoon is about ☐ a. 63 days. ☐ b. 75 days. ☐ c. 100 days. ☐ d. 116 days.	15	○
3.	When cornered, the raccoon seems ☐ a. to shake with fear. ☐ b. to become very aggressive. ☐ c. to withdraw. ☐ d. to stand very still.	15	○
4.	The phrase "black-masked eluder" gives the impression that the raccoon is good at ☐ a. robbing henhouses. ☐ b. hiding and playing tricks to escape hunting dogs. ☐ c. using disguises to trick predators. ☐ d. fighting off its enemies.	15	○
5.	As used in this passage, <u>pelt</u> refers to ☐ a. a large rodent. ☐ b. the claws of an animal. ☐ c. the action of beating something with a club. ☐ d. the skin of a furry animal.	15	○

6. Main Idea

	Answer	Score
Mark the main idea	M	10
Mark the statement that is a detail	D	5
Mark the statement that is too narrow	N	5
Mark the statement that is too broad	B	5

a. Raccoon skins were often made into hats.

b. Raccoons have many interesting characteristics.

c. We know some things about raccoons.

d. Raccoons eat meat and vegetables as humans do.

Total Comprehension Score
(Add your scores and enter the total on the graph on page 103.)

Categories of Comprehension Questions

No. 1: Subject Matter	No. 4: Clarifying Devices
No. 2: Supporting Details	No. 5: Vocabulary in Context
No. 3: Conclusion	No. 6: Main Idea

10. The Spring Peeper

The spring peeper is a common miniature frog belonging to the tree frog family. Its home covers the eastern part of North America from Canada to Florida. The peeper's body is a little less than one inch (about 2.5 centimeters) long; it is a trim little creature possessing rather long legs. Its toes are not webbed like those of the water frogs, but each toe has a small suction disk at the end which makes the peeper an inefficient swimmer but an excellent climber.

The peepers' diminutive size and lackluster color make them extremely difficult to see. Even if one is cheerfully calling just a short distance from you, you will be lucky if you can find it. In the daytime they usually call from under a leaf or floating twig, but after dark they scramble out onto grasses or stones.

Only the male peepers call. To do this the frog leans over backward and forces air into its throat cavity until the throat enlarges like a big bubble — the frog looks like a child chewing bubble gum! The call is produced with the mouth tightly closed; consequently, the bubble swells to a larger size with every "peep." The bubble finally collapses, leaving an empty bag of skin under the frog's throat.

If you walk near a swamp at night with a flashlight, you may be able to see these songsters. They do not seem to be afraid of the flashlight's rays; frequently, you can even pick them up.

In early spring, the peeper's eggs are deposited one at a time and usually are fastened to vegetation in the water. Peepers hatch after approximately one week. For the first few months they exist as tadpoles. By June they leave the water to exist on land as young frogs.

During the summer the peeper lives on the ground or in low bushes and vines. It doesn't usually climb very high. Each one lives by itself, and they never gather in groups except during the mating season in the spring. They feed upon tiny insects, spiders, small snails and worms. They are usually silent during the summer, but when one does call, its voice is discordant and insectlike — not at all like the harmonious spring song.

Peepers have many enemies — various fish, snakes, birds, skunks, foxes and other animals.

When frosty weather approaches, the peeper searches for a comfortable place on the forest floor where it can burrow down under leaves and mosses. There it hibernates, sleeping peacefully until the March sun melts the snow and the ice disappears from the ponds. Then all the peepers awake and hurry to the nearest marsh or swamp to begin their welcome spring chorus for another year.

_____ ? _____

	Possible Score	Your Score

1. The spring peeper is a

   ☐ a. frog.
   ☐ b. snake.
   ☐ c. toad.
   ☐ d. fish.   15   ○

2. The peeper's body is usually

   ☐ a. as big as a grain of salt.
   ☐ b. ¼ inch (about .6 centimeters) long.
   ☐ c. less than 1 inch (about 2.5 centimeters) long.
   ☐ d. from 6–7 inches (15.2–17.8 centimeters).   15   ○

3. A baby peeper spends the first few months of its life

   ☐ a. underground.
   ☐ b. inside a hollow tree.
   ☐ c. buried under leaves and moss.
   ☐ d. in the water.   15   ○

4. "Frosty weather" is

   ☐ a. rainy.
   ☐ b. cold.
   ☐ c. cloudy.
   ☐ d. windy.   15   ○

5. Peepers are <u>trim</u> little creatures. This means they are

   ☐ a. unfriendly.
   ☐ b. cheerful.
   ☐ c. thin.
   ☐ d. brightly colored.   15   ○

6. Main Idea

	Answer	Score
Mark the main idea	M	10
Mark the statement that is a detail	D	5
Mark the statement that is too narrow	N	5
Mark the statement that is too broad	B	5

a. Peepers have suction disks on their toes for climbing trees.

b. Certain frogs live more on land than in the water.

c. Spring peepers are small tree frogs with a spring song.

d. Spring peepers hibernate underground in the winter.

Total Comprehension Score
(Add your scores and enter the total on the graph on page 103.)

Categories of Comprehension Questions

No. 1: Subject Matter	No. 4: Clarifying Devices
No. 2: Supporting Details	No. 5: Vocabulary in Context
No. 3: Conclusion	No. 6: Main Idea

11. Under and Above Ground

Cicadas (sih KAY dahs), certainly the noisiest members of the insect world, exist in many varieties. No matter which variety they are, however, the males are the ones that produce all the "singing" noise. A few females can sing, but usually they are busy laying eggs by the thousands, so they let the males show off their singing.

While the male is vibrating his muscles in the treetops, the female is busy on the underside of a tree limb where she excavates two holes using the sharply pointed tube (*ovipositor*) that protrudes from the back of her body. In each of the holes she deposits six to eight fertile eggs. Then she selects another spot and does it all over again, and again, and again.

In a few weeks the eggs hatch, and little, black, antlike nymphs struggle out and drop to the ground. The moment they land they begin to dig into the soil with their strong, overdeveloped front legs that resemble tiny lobster claws and with their sharp, beaklike noses that help them to poke their way through.

Underground they eventually locate a tree root where they burrow a little hollow nest, stab their pointed beaks into the root and settle down to suck the sap. There they remain, making the nest larger as they grow.

The duration of their period in the ground changes with the variety of cicada they are. For example, the most common variety is the *harvester fly* which takes two years to develop underground, but another species, the *periodical cicada*, stays in the ground for seventeen years!

Finally the time arrives when they dig their way up to the surface and scramble to the nearest tree or bush. After climbing the tree as far as they can, they rest and prepare to shed the thick skin that encloses everything but their feet. As the air dries their skin, they wriggle about inside until the skin opens down the back and they are free.

They now begin to live their adult life, and in a very short time they search for a mate. Soon after they begin their egg laying, or, if they are males, they join a combo of noisy serenaders in a treetop.

Cicadas do not have a lengthy adult life. They live only about two weeks unless something kills them even sooner. They have many enemies, such as birds, which consider a juicy cicada a tasty snack. A single bird may eat thousands upon thousands of cicadas every year. This is an excellent example of the way nature balances out the populations of its various creatures.

_____ **?** _____

	Possible Score	Your Score

1. The cicadas are

    ☐ a. plants.
    ☐ b. mammals.
    ☐ c. insects.
    ☐ d. reptiles.

    (15)   ○

2. The cicada nymph spends its time

    ☐ a. under leaves.
    ☐ b. underground.
    ☐ c. in the air.
    ☐ d. in water.

    (15)   ○

3. After the cicada nymph builds a nest, it

    ☐ a. searches for food to store during winter.
    ☐ b. starts to care for its young.
    ☐ c. begins looking for a mate.
    ☐ d. stays there until it reaches adulthood.

    (15)   ○

4. The second paragraph talks about

    ☐ a. the reproduction of cicadas.
    ☐ b. how cicadas feed their young.
    ☐ c. the cicada's nest.
    ☐ d. cicada nymphs.

    (15)   ○

5. A <u>vibrating</u> muscle

    ☐ a. does not receive much oxygen.
    ☐ b. is flexed.
    ☐ c. moves back and forth.
    ☐ d. has totally collapsed.

    (15)   ○

6. Main Idea

	Answer	Score
Mark the main idea	M	(10)
Mark the statement that is a detail	D	(5)
Mark the statement that is too narrow	N	(5)
Mark the statement that is too broad	B	(5)

a. The periodical cicada stays underground for 17 years.

b. Cicadas change their habitat as they grow up.

c. Cicadas' life cycle includes stages above and below ground.

d. Cicada nymphs live underground and exist on tree sap.

Total Comprehension Score
(Add your scores and enter the total on the graph on page 103.)

Categories of Comprehension Questions

No. 1: Subject Matter	No. 4: Clarifying Devices
No. 2: Supporting Details	No. 5: Vocabulary in Context
No. 3: Conclusion	No. 6: Main Idea

12. Leave Them Alone!

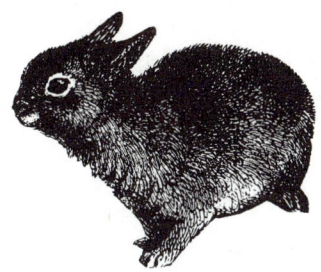

Look but don't touch is good advice when spring approaches. Spring is the season when wild creatures are busy replenishing their kind. It's also that time of year when children — and some adults — can't resist the urge to adopt a cuddly, cute, apparently helpless baby animal and take it home. But yielding to this temptation poses many problems for both the person and the animal.

In the first place, there is no such thing as a "pet permit." Removal of protected game birds, game animals or furbearing animals from the wild is against the law except during the legal open seasons. Even then they must, under law and regulations, be disposed of within certain time limits.

Secondly, the babies almost certainly aren't abandoned. Mother deer or rabbit is probably either nearby watching the whole thing with apprehension or out searching for food. The urge to pet or handle these young animals should be resisted. Touching them in any way can leave behind human scent that might upset the mother enough to cause her to abandon her young.

Virtually all wild animal babies grow up with a complete set of wild instincts and are frustrated if kept in captivity. They often become mischievous or even dangerous. Unless innoculated they can carry rabies, distemper and other diseases.

Persons adopting wild youngsters will invariably grow tired of them after they have outgrown the cuddly stage. Then it's a problem of knowing what to do with them. Simply killing the animals because they are no longer wanted is a cruel act, and many zoos will refuse to take them since they are already overstocked with most native species. Returning the adopted youngsters to the woods is not the solution since they are no longer equipped for survival in the wild.

The best way to avoid the problem is to leave wild animals in their natural habitat where they belong. Wild creatures have a better chance of survival if they are left alone — they get along better without a "helping hand." The best thing to do if you find wild baby animals is to take a quick look — then tiptoe quietly away.

?

| | Possible Score | Your Score |

1. What would be another good title for this passage?

   ☐ a. Wild Animals Don't Make Good Pets
   ☐ b. Dangerous Zoo Animals
   ☐ c. Snakes Are Not for Touching
   ☐ d. Be Careful, It Bites!

   (15)   ◯

2. Most animal babies are born in the

   ☐ a. summer.
   ☐ b. fall.
   ☐ c. winter.
   ☐ d. spring.

   (15)   ◯

3. If a pet animal is returned to its natural environment, it will most likely

   ☐ a. look for a home.
   ☐ b. not survive.
   ☐ c. seek a nest near humans.
   ☐ d. seek a mate.

   (15)   ◯

4. This author feels that most baby animals are

   ☐ a. cute and cuddly.
   ☐ b. homely and repulsive.
   ☐ c. quarrelsome and independent.
   ☐ d. diseased and weak.

   (15)   ◯

5. Another word for <u>innoculated</u> is

   ☐ a. diseased.
   ☐ b. nursed.
   ☐ c. groomed.
   ☐ d. vaccinated.

   (15)   ◯

6. Main Idea

	Answer	Score
Mark the main idea	M	(10)
Mark the statement that is a detail	D	(5)
Mark the statement that is too narrow	N	(5)
Mark the statement that is too broad	B	(5)

a. A baby animal found by itself is probably not abandoned.

b. An attempt to be kind to an animal may really be cruel.

c. Wild animals raised as pets may become dangerous.

d. Wild baby animals should be left in their natural habitat.

Total Comprehension Score
(Add your scores and enter the total on the graph on page 103.)

Categories of Comprehension Questions

No. 1: Subject Matter	No. 4: Clarifying Devices
No. 2: Supporting Details	No. 5: Vocabulary in Context
No. 3: Conclusion	No. 6: Main Idea

13. Moving Rocks for Locks

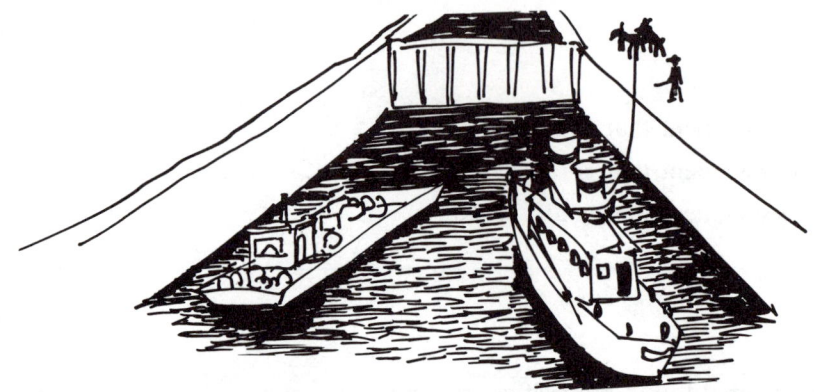

Its Revolutionary War had been over only a very few years when the United States was forced to find relief for its growing pains by expanding westward. But the journey then, across the hazy line of the western frontier, was long, tedious and very expensive.

Fortunately, in the early 1800s, the United States was gripped in a passion for canals patterned after the successful artificial waterways of Europe. The cross-state survey of the proposed canal route through New York was made by two lawyers, but lawyers who had the vision and zeal of engineers. Their survey proved to be more than adequate, and it was decided to start digging at a spot near Rome, New York.

As could be expected of a project of this size, there was a strong opposition which jeered and called the project to build the Erie Canal *Clinton's Folly* (after DeWitt Clinton, the canal's sponsor and Governor of New York).

The project was backbreaking work with pick, shovel and wheelbarrow, but the laborers worked enthusiastically, having pride in being part of a great dream. Rocks had to be drilled by hand and blown out of the soil with black powder. The powerful equipment of today was, of course, not known.

A total of seventy-two locks were built to achieve a lift of 500 feet (about 152 meters) between the Hudson River and Lake Erie. Each lock was 12 feet (about 3.7 meters) wide and 90 feet (about 27.4 meters) long, and the average lock lift was about 7 feet (about 2.1 meters).

On November 4, 1825, eight years after the first spadeful of soil was turned, the great canal was completed. What was jeered at as "Clinton's Folly" turned out to be a bonanza for the state of New York, as well as for the United States. The way west was truly opened. Produce and merchandise that used to spend a month in transit now moved from New York City to Buffalo in ten days. In the first year of operation, the canal earned more than a half million dollars in tolls. Long after the railroads were built, the Erie was still making money and did not reach the peak of its tonnage until 1880. Its most triumphant creation, however, was modern New York City, which otherwise might have been just another seaport.

?

	Possible Score	Your Score

1. What would be another good title for this passage?

   ☐ a. The Hudson River Overflows
   ☐ b. Clinton's Folly
   ☐ c. Canals of Europe
   ☐ d. New York and Its Problems

   (15)   ◯

2. The Erie Canal was finished in

   ☐ a. 1776.
   ☐ b. 1810.
   ☐ c. 1820.
   ☐ d. 1825.

   (15)   ◯

3. The Erie Canal

   ☐ a. helped with westward expansion.
   ☐ b. was unsuccessful.
   ☐ c. has recently been replaced.
   ☐ d. was never finished.

   (15)   ◯

4. When a country has "growing pains," it means the country is

   ☐ a. starting to decline.
   ☐ b. at war.
   ☐ c. beginning to develop.
   ☐ d. at a standstill.

   (15)   ◯

5. To jeer means

   ☐ a. to cheer.
   ☐ b. to complete.
   ☐ c. to announce.
   ☐ d. to ridicule.

   (15)   ◯

6. Main Idea

	Answer	Score
Mark the main idea	M	10
Mark the statement that is a detail	D	5
Mark the statement that is too narrow	N	5
Mark the statement that is too broad	B	5

a. Big projects are often worth the effort they take.

b. There is a 500-foot (152-meter) lift between Lake Erie and the Hudson.

c. The Erie Canal was responsible for the growth of New York City.

d. The Erie Canal proved beneficial to the United States.

Total Comprehension Score
(Add your scores and enter the total on the graph on page 103.)

Categories of Comprehension Questions

No. 1: Subject Matter	No. 4: Clarifying Devices
No. 2: Supporting Details	No. 5: Vocabulary in Context
No. 3: Conclusion	No. 6: Main Idea

14. Salt Water Bait Too

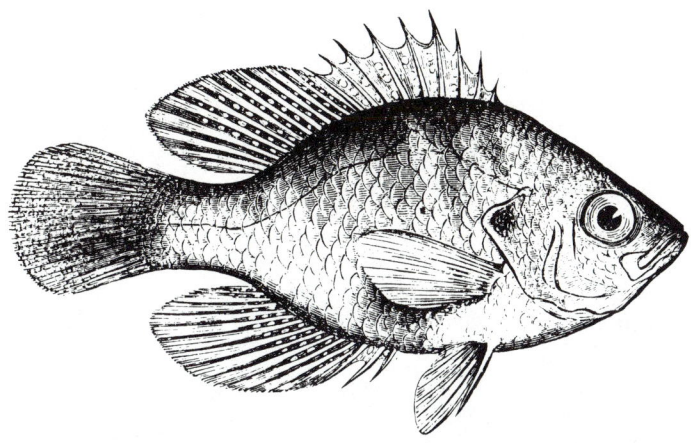

For years manufacturers offered selected artificial saltwater lures that looked artificial. Then the manufacturers graduated to really impressive saltwater lures. Coastal fishers quickly bought the realistic-looking eels, squid, baitfish and imitation cut bait. They discovered that they not only worked beautifully but were much more durable than the real thing. A fresh balao baitfish only lasts until the first serious strike; a vinyl plastic imitation costs twice as much, but it lasts and lasts — maybe all day, maybe all week.

Today, the sporting goods stores can offer many saltwater lures, from insects a half inch (about 1.3 centimeters) long to flying fish sixteen inches (about 40.6 centimeters) long. They're available in a rainbow of colors, but the natural and black worms still are the favorites and still catch the most bass.

Plenty of fishers, however, still don't use artificial lures. This is because not everyone has discovered the secret of catching fish with them. Many fishers have tried, failed and gone back to their natural lures.

What's the secret? You can get it into one sentence: plastic lures, especially the worms, must be fished as slowly as you can move them and still keep them wiggling. That means agonizingly slow, as slow as you can possibly revolve a reel handle, so slow that you can detect the lead head sliding, bouncing and scraping along the bottom, so slow that you can feel every rock and log and twig — and every fish that takes the lure inquisitively into its mouth. Then you wait patiently, remaining lightly in touch without overtightening the line, until you can't endure the situation any more or until the fish swims away with it. Then pull it, hard, and pull it again to make sure.

It's the simplest secret in fishing. It's been printed a thousand times in books, magazines and on the labels of the worm packages. I doubted it myself until a couple of years ago, but now I've seen the plastic light. It's doubled my catch on large-mouth bass, and it can double yours. Try it.

?

	Possible Score	Your Score

1. This passage centers on

   ☐ a. live bait fishing.
   ☐ b. the making of metal lures.
   ☐ c. plastic lures.
   ☐ d. homemade lures.

   15

2. The secret of using the new lures is

   ☐ a. to move the lures as slowly as possible.
   ☐ b. to jerk the lure up and down.
   ☐ c. to make sure the line is loose.
   ☐ d. to keep the lure from touching bottom.

   15

3. From this passage we can conclude that

   ☐ a. live bait is quite inexpensive.
   ☐ b. some imitation lures are better than live bait.
   ☐ c. large-mouth fish are easy to catch.
   ☐ d. imitation lures are still not perfected.

   15

4. What does the author mean by the phrase, "now I've seen the plastic light"?

   ☐ a. He now knows how to use plastic lures.
   ☐ b. Imitation lures are not as good as live bait.
   ☐ c. The author finds vinyl fishing poles the best.
   ☐ d. It's a good idea to take a lantern for night fishing.

   15

5. Another word for <u>inquisitive</u> is

   ☐ a. vicious.
   ☐ b. lazy.
   ☐ c. curious.
   ☐ d. fierce.

   15

6. Main Idea

	Answer	Score
Mark the main idea	M	(10)
Mark the statement that is a detail	D	(5)
Mark the statement that is too narrow	N	(5)
Mark the statement that is too broad	B	(5)

a. The narrator doubled his catch using plastic lures slowly.

b. Modern methods of fishing must be used correctly.

c. Realistic-looking artifical baits are made of vinyl plastic.

d. Plastic lures can increase your catch when fished very slowly.

Total Comprehension Score
(Add your scores and enter the total on the graph on page 103.)

Categories of Comprehension Questions

No. 1: Subject Matter	No. 4: Clarifying Devices
No. 2: Supporting Details	No. 5: Vocabulary in Context
No. 3: Conclusion	No. 6: Main Idea

15. Snow As an Insulator

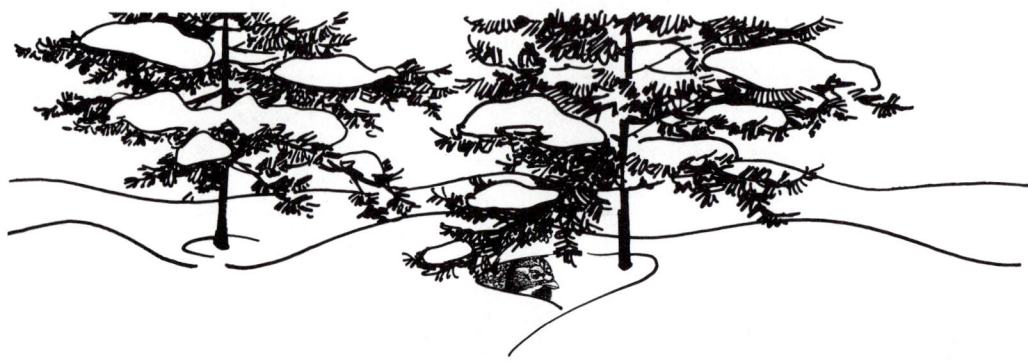

The snow *surface* may become extremely cold on a clear winter night, but below the surface the temperature may be many degrees warmer. This is because a snow *blanket* contains a lot of air, which is an effective insulator against heat *conduction*. For this reason, many small mammals live quite comfortably beneath a snow cover in winter, despite a climate above the snow severe enough to kill them. *Shrews*, tiny mammals whose metabolism is so high that they are almost never still, make tunnels under the snow when it is only an inch or two deep rather than dart about above the snow. Part of this may be for protection from predators, but part of it may be that the climate beneath the snow is more hospitable.

Some animals make use of snowbanks for protection in heavy snowstorms. Grouse are known to fly from tree perches directly into a snow bank and remain there for the duration of a storm. If a glaze of ice happens to cover the snow after the storm and prevents the birds from digging out of their natural igloos, they may be trapped so long that they starve, suffocate or become prey for foxes and other predators that walk on top of the crust. But a snowbank has probably saved the lives of many birds and other animals in severe weather.

Plants whose tender parts would be killed by extreme cold often survive if they are insulated from the severe climate by an air-filled snow blanket. If a snowfall covers a boxwood hedge, for example, its owner may be tempted to knock off the snow and thus keep branches from breaking. However, it may be wise to leave a snow cover on such plants if only to protect them from extremes of temperature which might otherwise kill the plants.

Besides safeguarding small mammals and some birds, a snow cover protects untold numbers of insects, worms, snails and many other small creatures in the soil. Without the snow blanket, soil temperatures in winter would plunge low enough to kill many of the organisms in it. Snow, however, prevents this. The lowest temperatures are at the top of the snow cover, not at its base.

?

	Possible Score	Your Score

1. What would be another good title for this passage?

   ☐ a. How Snow Forms
   ☐ b. Snow, A Blanket of Protection
   ☐ c. Weather Patterns of Snow Storms
   ☐ d. Snowy Regions of the North

   (15)

2. Which of the following birds are known to fly into snowbanks?

   ☐ a. Pigeons
   ☐ b. Pheasant
   ☐ c. Quails
   ☐ d. Grouse

   (15)

3. We can conclude from this passage that

   ☐ a. air is a good insulator.
   ☐ b. water conducts heat.
   ☐ c. a snow cover causes the ground to freeze.
   ☐ d. snow is a deadly killer.

   (15)

4. A "snow blanket" is a

   ☐ a. woven cloth.
   ☐ b. violent storm.
   ☐ c. covering of snow.
   ☐ d. type of tunnel.

   (15)

5. A bird might <u>suffocate</u> if there is a lack of

   ☐ a. air.
   ☐ b. food.
   ☐ c. water.
   ☐ d. heat.

   (15)

6. Main Idea

	Answer	Score
Mark the main idea	M	10
Mark the statement that is a detail	D	5
Mark the statement that is too narrow	N	5
Mark the statement that is too broad	B	5

a. Any material that traps air is a good insulator.

b. A glaze of ice can trap a grouse inside a snow bank.

c. Snow contains air, so it insulates against cold.

d. A bird will bury itself in a snow bank when it's cold.

Total Comprehension Score
(Add your scores and enter the
total on the graph on page 103.)

Categories of Comprehension Questions

No. 1: Subject Matter	No. 4: Clarifying Devices
No. 2: Supporting Details	No. 5: Vocabulary in Context
No. 3: Conclusion	No. 6: Main Idea

16. That Butterfly Is Really a Clam!

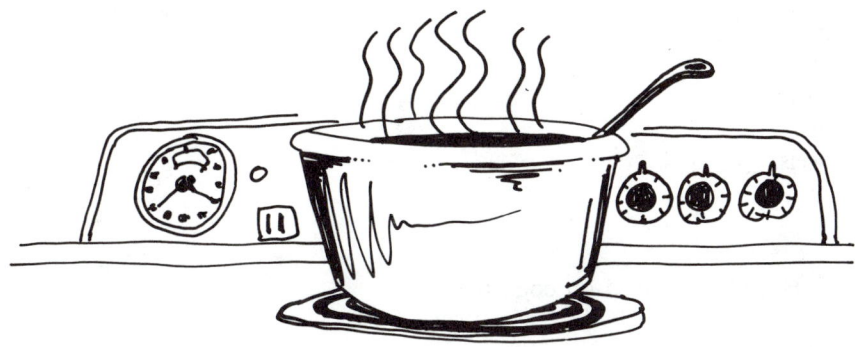

Coquinas subsist on miniature plants and animals of the ocean called *plankton*. When a coquina feeds, its shell is almost closed; the only things sticking out are two slender tubes — like tiny snorkels.

Through one of these tubes the coquina draws sea water containing plankton into the shell. At the interior of the shell the water passes over the animal's gills, and the plankton are caught in an adhesive material on the gills. The gills have tiny hairs that push the food into the animal's mouth. Under a microscope the coquina's gills resemble a forest of waving hairs — all swaying in the same direction.

Water and waste materials are excreted by the animal through the other tube, so while the animal feeds, water simultaneously flows into one tube, over the gills and out the other tube.

Because shore birds and crabs feed on these little sea animals, coquinas are consequently excellent diggers. A specially developed muscle called the *foot* is the coquina's "instrument" for digging and burrowing. The coquina pushes its fleshy foot into the sand, and once in the sand, the tip of the foot enlarges and works like an anchor. Then the remainder of the foot shortens which pulls the coquina's shell down under the sand. The entire digging activity takes only a second: pushing, swelling, pulling, and now you see them, now you don't!

Birds and crabs aren't the only creatures that eat coquinas; people do, too! Coquina soup is a favorite among people living along our southern coastlines. Coquina hunters use a shallow sieve and a little shovel. After scooping the sand and coquinas into the sieve, they allow the water to wash out the sand, leaving only the coquinas. They keep the coquinas alive in a bucket of ocean water until it's time to cook them.

One thing is certain — even if you never taste coquina soup, you can enjoy the beauty of this little animal's butterfly-shaped shell. The coquina is truly the most beautiful "butterfly" living in our sandy beaches.

_____ ? _____

| | Possible Score | Your Score |

1. The coquinas are

   ☐ a. butterflies.
   ☐ b. clams.
   ☐ c. mussels.
   ☐ d. crabs.   15   ○

2. Which of the following feed on coquinas?

   ☐ a. Sea lions
   ☐ b. Shore birds and crabs
   ☐ c. Starfish
   ☐ d. Mussels   15   ○

3. The writer suggests that people along our southern coastlines find coquinas

   ☐ a. tough.
   ☐ b. tasty.
   ☐ c. delicate.
   ☐ d. very active.   15   ○

4. The last paragraph compares the coquina to

   ☐ a. the most beautiful butterfly.
   ☐ b. a graceful bird.
   ☐ c. the seashore.
   ☐ d. a green forest.   15   ○

5. The coquina's <u>fleshy</u> foot is

   ☐ a. bony.
   ☐ b. soft.
   ☐ c. hard.
   ☐ d. liquidy.   15   ○

6. Main Idea

	Answer	Score
Mark the main idea	M	10
Mark the statement that is a detail	D	5
Mark the statement that is too narrow	N	5
Mark the statement that is too broad	B	5

a. A coquina can dig itself out of sight in a second.

b. The coquina is one of many small sea animals.

c. The coquina captures plankton with its gills.

d. The coquina is a plankton-feeding sea creature.

Total Comprehension Score
(Add your scores and enter the
total on the graph on page 103.)

Categories of Comprehension Questions

No. 1: Subject Matter	No. 4: Clarifying Devices
No. 2: Supporting Details	No. 5: Vocabulary in Context
No. 3: Conclusion	No. 6: Main Idea

71

17. Hippie of the Feathered World

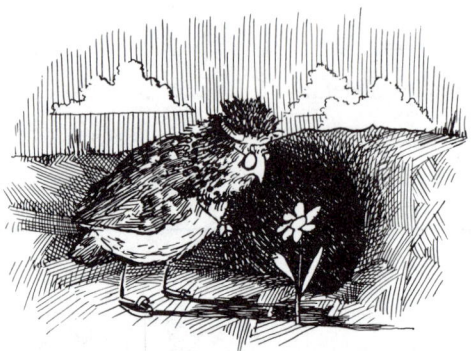

I could hardly believe my eyes. One moment my horse had reared up as an owl rose in front of us, a still struggling mouse in its talons, and the next moment, bird and mouse had disappeared as though the earth had swallowed them. Amazingly, it had. I had come upon a hippie of the feathered world, a defiant denizen of the bird establishment who prefers to live underground. It was a burrowing owl, one of the most unusual of over 500 different kinds of owls in the world. Aside from its quick exits from the sight of people, it is disappearing in another way. With the increase of farming and the gradual disappearance of grasslands and prairie-dog towns, the burrowing owl is indeed becoming a rarer bird each year.

A beneficial bird, brownish-barred in color, the burrowing owl eats small rodents, such as field mice, and many varieties of insects. If there are enough, it can live on grasshoppers alone. The burrowing owl measures from eight to ten inches (20.3 to 25.4 centimeters) in height, has a stubby tail, a round head which can swivel nearly full circle, and piercing yellow eyes. Both sexes look alike. Their long legs are well adapted to hunting on the ground; however, they are equally proficient at hunting from the air. They dart up to snatch passing insects and swoop low or hover over a field to seize unsuspecting mice.

A distinguishing characteristic of this small owl is its continuous bobbing motion caused by a quick bending of the legs. It is often seen bobbing on fence posts or near the earthen mound of its burrow.

For their homes, burrowing owls will drive prairie dogs or other rodents from their burrows and take over. Though they can dig fine tunnels, usually they prefer an abandoned burrow, especially an old badger hole. In Florida, they must dig their own holes because none of their neighbors dig any to suit them. The owls might do a little remodeling of a "captured" hole before moving in, but as a rule they get right to work collecting small chips of cow manure to line a nest. The female lays from five to seven white eggs, and both parents may participate in incubating them. When one is on the nest, the other does sentry duty on a rock or post near the hole opening.

?

| | Possible Score | Your Score |

1. This passage is about the

   ☐ a. burrowing owl.
   ☐ b. screech owl.
   ☐ c. barn owl.
   ☐ d. great horned owl.

   (15)

2. The owl in this passage lives

   ☐ a. on rocky ledges.
   ☐ b. in cedar trees.
   ☐ c. in caves.
   ☐ d. underground.

   (15)

3. According to this passage, an increase in farming sometimes means that

   ☐ a. there will be more food for everyone in the United States.
   ☐ b. fewer people are working in factories.
   ☐ c. wild animals are eating more and more of the farmer's crops.
   ☐ d. certain forms of wildlife lose their homes.

   (15)

4. What was the author of this passage doing when the owl appeared?

   ☐ a. Fishing
   ☐ b. Horseback riding
   ☐ c. Hunting
   ☐ d. Playing golf

   (15)

5. If an owl is a <u>proficient</u> hunter, this means it

   ☐ a. is a good hunter.
   ☐ b. is just learning to hunt.
   ☐ c. lacks hunting skills.
   ☐ d. likes to hunt in groups.

   (15)

6. Main Idea

	Answer	Score
Mark the main idea	M	10
Mark the statement that is a detail	D	5
Mark the statement that is too narrow	N	5
Mark the statement that is too broad	B	5

a. Burrowing owls can live on a diet of grasshoppers alone.

b. The burrowing owl can dig a fine tunnel for a home.

c. Burrowing owls have habits different from other owls.

d. Burrowing owls are owls which live in burrows.

Total Comprehension Score
(Add your scores and enter the total on the graph on page 103.)

Categories of Comprehension Questions

No. 1: Subject Matter	No. 4: Clarifying Devices
No. 2: Supporting Details	No. 5: Vocabulary in Context
No. 3: Conclusion	No. 6: Main Idea

18. The Most Ferocious Animal in the Woods

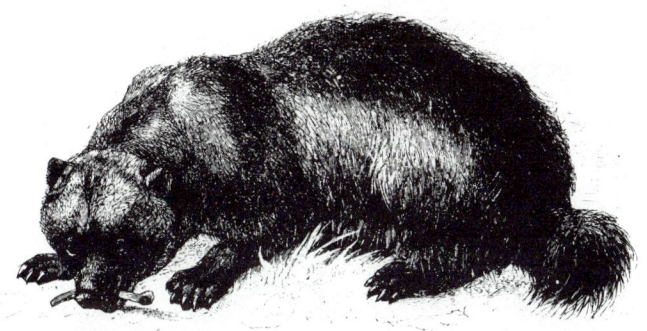

It's one of the most savage and relentless battlers of the wild, and for its size, it's the most ferocious animal in the world. For its size, no living creature can match the wolverine.

Squat and bearlike, seldom weighing more than forty pounds (about 18.1 kilograms), largest of the weasel family, it is a terror to all other animals. A wolverine in California's Sierra Nevadas once came upon two bears devouring a fresh carcass. Every hair bristling, it hoisted its tail and charged. As the little marauder leaped between them, the bears fled.

Once in the north woods a wolverine forced a pack of hungry wolves from a meal. After nonchalantly consuming all it desired of the kill, the wolverine sprayed the remains with its evil-smelling scent so that the wolves would not return to eat.

Utterly fearless, it neither asks nor gives quarter; it can and will fight anything, anywhere. As it rushes into combat, it growls and grunts, and no matter what the odds, it never gives ground — it is victory or death. Its jaws and teeth are immensely strong, capable of crushing large bones and tearing the toughest flesh. The heavy-clawed paws are also devastating, death-dealing instruments.

Even an entire team of Alaskan huskies is no match for it. On one occasion, a wolverine encountered a whole pack of these powerful dogs and swept through them like a tornado, leaving behind a trail of torn flesh.

Yet another time, one was known to have killed a polar bear — quite a feat when the great white bear may weigh more than 1,000 pounds (about 453.6 kilograms) and is regarded as the master of the polar world.

The wolverine is driven by a ravenous appetite to waging a never-ending campaign for food. It plods its leisurely way through the forest, feeding on anything edible. It is so skilled a hunter that it rarely is found in a starved condition; however, its voracious appetite sometimes is the wolverine's undoing. When pressed for food, it will attack even a porcupine. Dead wolverines have been found, their insides loaded with quills.

_____ **?** _____

	Possible Score	Your Score

1. This passage is about the wolverine and its

   ☐ a. young.
   ☐ b. ferocious nature.
   ☐ c. appearance.
   ☐ d. nesting habits.

   (15) ◯

2. The wolverine weighs about

   ☐ a. 10 pounds (about 4.54 kilograms).
   ☐ b. 40 pounds (about 18.1 kilograms).
   ☐ c. 80 pounds (about 36.3 kilograms).
   ☐ d. 1 ton (about .9 tonnes).

   (15) ◯

3. Which of the following is most likely true?

   ☐ a. Sometimes small animals are the most vicious.
   ☐ b. Even shy animals get along with the wolverine.
   ☐ c. Many animals are fussy about what they eat.
   ☐ d. Wolverines travel with wild dog packs.

   (15) ◯

4. The wolverine never "gives ground." This means it

   ☐ a. lives in the burrow alone.
   ☐ b. never gives up.
   ☐ c. sprays the ground with its scent.
   ☐ d. will not paw the ground before a fight.

   (15) ◯

5. As used in this passage, campaign means a

   ☐ a. feast.
   ☐ b. home.
   ☐ c. trail.
   ☐ d. search.

   (15) ◯

6. Main Idea

	Answer	Score
Mark the main idea	M	10
Mark the statement that is a detail	D	5
Mark the statement that is too narrow	N	5
Mark the statement that is too broad	B	5

a. The wolverine is the largest member of the weasel family.

b. A wolverine can drive bears away from their kill.

c. The wolverine is the most ferocious animal for its size.

d. Size is not the only proof of an animal's fighting ability.

Total Comprehension Score
(Add your scores and enter the
total on the graph on page 103.)

Categories of Comprehension Questions

No. 1: Subject Matter	No. 4: Clarifying Devices
No. 2: Supporting Details	No. 5: Vocabulary in Context
No. 3: Conclusion	No. 6: Main Idea

19. The Buffalo Hunters

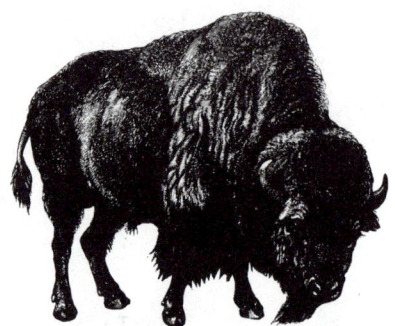

Throughout the thousands of years before white people settled on this continent, North American Indians roamed far and wide over what is today Canada, the United States and Mexico.

For hundreds of years, the Indians depended on hunting and fishing for their food. To improve their skill at catching animals and fish, the Indians would observe the daily and seasonal habits of the game they were after. In this way, they acquired more and more knowledge about the wildlife around them.

Among the Plains Indians, hunting scouts were known as *wolves*. In their dances and when following a trail, each scout wore an entire wolfskin that fitted over his head and back with the wolfskin's forelegs fastened to the scout's arms. To make them appear authentic, the ears of the wolfskin were coated with clay. When the clay dried, it became hard and made the triangular-shaped ears stand erect.

During the centuries before they acquired horses, Plains Indians used these wolfskin coverings when they hunted the buffalo. By observing carefully, the Indians had noticed that a few wolves moving close to a herd of buffalo did not frighten the big animals. They decided to put what they had learned to good use. The Indians would put on the wolfskins and slowly approach the herd on their hands and knees. When they got close enough, their well-aimed arrows would bring down a few of the grass-eating buffalo before the herd stampeded.

When horses first arrived in the western regions, they were few in number. But even then they altered the buffalo hunters' methods. Selected hunters would mount their horses and travel to where the buffalo were feeding. At a safe distance the riders would camouflage themselves with buffalo robes, lean forward over their horses' necks, and, as the horses grazed, the riders would slowly move in among the herd.

During such hunts, the younger Indians were often allowed to watch at a distance. In this way, they learned the skills that would be expected of them when they grew older.

_____ **?** _____

	Possible Score	Your Score

1. What would be another good title for this passage?

   ☐ a. Learning To Hunt Buffalo
   ☐ b. Uses of the Buffalo Hide
   ☐ c. The Dying Out of the Buffalo
   ☐ d. The Buffalo — a Fearsome Enemy

   (15)   ◯

2. Before they had horses, the Indians would hunt buffalo using

   ☐ a. poisoned meat.
   ☐ b. wolfskin coverings.
   ☐ c. bear traps.
   ☐ d. guns.

   (15)   ◯

3. Buffalo get their food by

   ☐ a. hunting.
   ☐ b. fighting.
   ☐ c. digging.
   ☐ d. grazing.

   (15)   ◯

4. The second paragraph tells us

   ☐ a. where the Indians lived.
   ☐ b. how Indians learned about animal habits.
   ☐ c. why the Indians hunted buffalo.
   ☐ d. how the Indians fished.

   (15)   ◯

5. If a wolf's ears are standing <u>erect</u>, they are

   ☐ a. tilted forward.
   ☐ b. pointed straight up.
   ☐ c. laying down flat.
   ☐ d. bent sideways.

   (15)   ◯

6. Main Idea

	Answer	Score
Mark the main idea	M	10
Mark the statement that is a detail	D	5
Mark the statement that is too narrow	N	5
Mark the statement that is too broad	B	5

a. Indians hunted the plains centuries before the settlers came.

b. The Indians improved their hunting by observing their game's habits.

c. The Indians hunted buffalo by imitating wolves.

d. The Indians put what they learned to good use.

Total Comprehension Score
(Add your scores and enter the total on the graph on page 103.)

Categories of Comprehension Questions

No. 1: Subject Matter	No. 4: Clarifying Devices
No. 2: Supporting Details	No. 5: Vocabulary in Context
No. 3: Conclusion	No. 6: Main Idea

20. Foxy Family

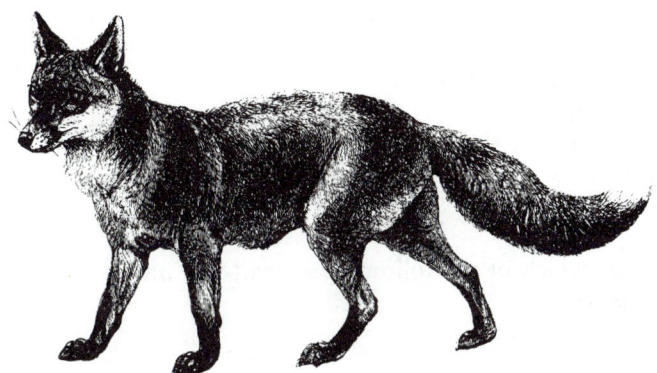

Red foxes breed in the late part of January or the early part of February, and five to eight pups are born about the middle of March. The pups' eyes, which open in nine days, are blue at the beginning, then gradually turn yellow within two months; the ears are sealed at birth but open soon afterward.

Both male and female devote themselves to the young. Initially, the female remains with her pups constantly while the male brings food to her. After several weeks the female can leave the pups for increasing lengths of time. Finally, she too resumes hunting.

At six weeks the pups venture out of the den and begin eating solid food. Previously fed regurgitated meat, they are now brought mice, voles, ground squirrels, rabbits and similar food.

As the pups grow older, the parents drop food farther and farther from the den, thus teaching them to hunt. But venturing farther from the safety of the den each day also increases their exposure to danger. The unseen, circling speck high in the sky can materialize within seconds into a plummeting eagle. In forested areas the bobcat, fisher, lynx and wolverine will quickly add a fox pup to their diet whenever possible. Bobcats and fishers take a pup only if the adult fox is not near, while lynx and wolverines will also kill adults. Large predators, such as the bear, mountain lion, coyote and wolf, do not ordinarily hunt foxes but will kill one if the opportunity arises. A fox is particularly <u>fearful</u> of the wolf and, in rural areas, of dogs.

As the pups mature, they follow their parents farther afield to hunt, and by summer all will be practicing what will become a lifelong habit of sleeping in the open.

By autumn the fox family will have separated. Most of the young will stay in the general area because danger lies in the unfamiliar. Others may move but stay close, while some may move long distances away.

_____ **?** _____

		Possible Score	Your Score

1. This passage is about

   ☐ a. photographing the red fox.
   ☐ b. red fox pups.
   ☐ c. the sly nature of the red fox.
   ☐ d. the fur of the red fox.   (15)   ◯

2. In rural areas, which of the following seems to be an enemy of the fox?

   ☐ a. The eagle
   ☐ b. The dog
   ☐ c. The bobcat
   ☐ d. The fisher   (15)   ◯

3. Red foxes breed in

   ☐ a. early summer.
   ☐ b. late fall.
   ☐ c. late winter.
   ☐ d. early spring.   (15)   ◯

4. The fourth paragraph discusses the

   ☐ a. natural enemies of the red fox.
   ☐ b. appearance of the red fox.
   ☐ c. nature of the red fox.
   ☐ d. hunting habits of the red fox.   (15)   ◯

5. The fox is <u>fearful</u> of the wolf. This means the fox

   ☐ a. will often hunt a wolf.
   ☐ b. and wolf are friends.
   ☐ c. lives near the wolf.
   ☐ d. is afraid of the wolf.   (15)   ◯

6. Main Idea

	Answer	Score
Mark the main idea	M	10
Mark the statement that is a detail	D	5
Mark the statement that is too narrow	N	5
Mark the statement that is too broad	B	5

a. Male and female foxes work together to raise their young.

b. Young animals often need care from both their parents.

c. An adult fox will chase some predators away from its pups.

d. Fox pups' eyes change color from blue to yellow after birth.

Total Comprehension Score
(Add your scores and enter the total on the graph on page 103.)

Categories of Comprehension Questions

No. 1: Subject Matter	No. 4: Clarifying Devices
No. 2: Supporting Details	No. 5: Vocabulary in Context
No. 3: Conclusion	No. 6: Main Idea

83

21. The Red Fox As a Hunter

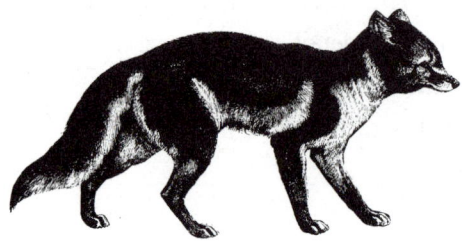

The red fox thrives on autumn's plenty — berries and fruits, numerous insects and all varieties of feathered and furred game. Red foxes consume about one pound (about .45 kilograms) of food a day, but when one catches more food than can be eaten, it buries the remainder. It digs a hole with its forelegs, drops in the surplus food and pushes dirt over it with its nose. This buried food will remain fresh a long time, but the fox will eat carrion as well as fresh food.

A fox will utilize whatever game is wounded or killed by hunters and then not found by them. In winter, every deer that has been shot and lost or that has died of starvation is a bonanza to the red fox.

The mainstay of the red fox in winter, however, is the cottontail rabbit, which provides sixty percent or more of its diet. But given proper habitat, the rabbit population will easily withstand the combined pressure of all predators — the proof of this is that they have been doing just that for millions of years.

The same holds true for the red fox in its relationship to other game species. It has been accused of extra-heavy predations of quail populations in some areas. Evidence has not fully supported this accusation. When the ring-neck pheasant population decreased nationally in the mid-1940s, accusing fingers were quickly pointed at the red fox. No one can say positively what caused the pheasants to decline in number, but it was not solely the red fox. On Ontario's Pelee Island — world famous for its pheasant hunting — the ring-neck population decreased correspondingly, but there are no foxes on Pelee.

Nearly every governmental body in the United States has set bounties at one time or another in attempts to control the red fox population, but with few exceptions, the controls have failed.

So it goes in the life of a red fox. Despite its simplistic existence, it's an enigma. It's been hunted and trapped, cursed and maligned. Yet, it somehow survives and survives well. The red fox is a cunning species, unafraid, but always alert — truly the living symbol of cleverness and intelligence.

?

	Possible Score	Your Score

1. The main topic of this passage is the red fox and its

   ☐ a. losing fight for survival.
   ☐ b. predatory habits.
   ☐ c. close relationship to the kit fox.
   ☐ d. wintering habits.

   (15) ○

2. The main food of the red fox in winter is

   ☐ a. fruit.
   ☐ b. the cottontail rabbit.
   ☐ c. buried carrion.
   ☐ d. the field mouse.

   (15) ○

3. At times the red fox

   ☐ a. has been hunted for a reward.
   ☐ b. will migrate southward.
   ☐ c. has been known to starve to death.
   ☐ d. will take more than one mate.

   (15) ○

4. The writer feels that the red fox is

   ☐ a. misunderstood.
   ☐ b. a rare species.
   ☐ c. quite a nuisance to farmers.
   ☐ d. overprotected.

   (15) ○

5. An <u>enigma</u> is

   ☐ a. a rodent.
   ☐ b. an enemy.
   ☐ c. a puzzle.
   ☐ d. a companion.

   (15) ○

6. Main Idea

	Answer	Score
Mark the main idea	M	10
Mark the statement that is a detail	D	5
Mark the statement that is too narrow	N	5
Mark the statement that is too broad	B	5

a. Foxes are balanced in their habits.

b. The red fox has often been hunted.

c. The red fox is not guilty of overhunting.

d. The red fox eats rabbits without wiping them out.

Total Comprehension Score
(Add your scores and enter the total on the graph on page 103.)

Categories of Comprehension Questions

No. 1: Subject Matter	No. 4: Clarifying Devices
No. 2: Supporting Details	No. 5: Vocabulary in Context
No. 3: Conclusion	No. 6: Main Idea

22. Pop-Out and Fall-Away Seeds

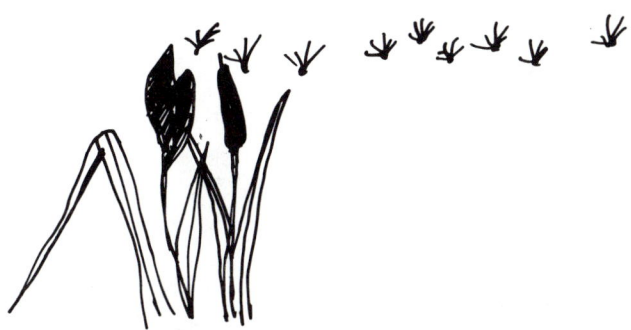

Witch hazel has developed a method to scatter its seeds which is not dependent upon birds, barbs or breezes. As it dries, the open-ended container slowly squeezes the seeds until they pop out, sometimes for a surprising distance. You can witness a witch hazel pop its seeds if you collect some of its branches bearing unopened fruit in September and keep them in a warm room. Occasionally, one will pop all the way across the room.

Jewelweed or touch-me-not is another example of a seed popper. In late summer its fruits hang like miniature cucumbers from the underside of its stems. They seem to bulge from the two or three oversized and nutritious seeds within the fruit. If you attempt to pick one of these fruits, you must do it carefully, for a ripe fruit will split open at a touch, scattering the seeds several inches away. If you can cup your hand around the touch-me-not fruit and capture the seeds as they pop out of their container, you will have a delicious treat tasting a little like black walnuts.

Some seeds are not edible, nor do they travel with the wind, nor do they have spines for adhering to fur or clothing. Their only means of scattering is to roll or tumble on a hillside. Osage orange, for example, produces a fruit the size of a baseball, lumpy and orangish yellow, and its juice is sticky white. Hardly any animal except young children take an interest in them. The fruits can roll quite far on sloping ground, but children can throw them even farther.

The coconut fruit is one of the world's largest seeds; it is heavy, almost impenetrable, and cannot be carried by wind or small animals. When it falls into water, however, it floats and may be washed or blown out to sea. Salt water appears to have minimal effect on it, and when it eventually washes up on a distant shore, only slightly scratched by the hazardous journey, the seed it contains may germinate. The coconut, almost the biggest and heaviest of seeds, may hold a record for distance traveled.

?

	Possible Score	Your Score

1. The seeds being discussed in this passage are

    ☐ a. witch hazel, jewelweed, osage orange, and coconut.
    ☐ b. milkweed and dandelion.
    ☐ c. burdocks.
    ☐ d. maple, oak, elm and sassafras.

    (15)

2. Which of the following is considered one of the biggest seeds in the world?

    ☐ a. The milkweed seed
    ☐ b. The elm seed
    ☐ c. The burdock seed
    ☐ d. The coconut seed

    (15)

3. From this passage, we can conclude that in order to germinate a seed

    ☐ a. needs lots of sunlight.
    ☐ b. must be dispersed.
    ☐ c. should be carried by the wind.
    ☐ d. cannot be soaked with water.

    (15)

4. In appearance, the touch-me-not seeds resemble

    ☐ a. crab apples.
    ☐ b. coconuts.
    ☐ c. black walnuts.
    ☐ d. small cucumbers.

    (15)

5. An <u>edible</u> seed is one that

    ☐ a. is poisonous.
    ☐ b. did not develop.
    ☐ c. can be eaten.
    ☐ d. will not germinate.

    (15)

6. Main Idea

	Answer	Score
Mark the main idea	M	10
Mark the statement that is a detail	D	5
Mark the statement that is too narrow	N	5
Mark the statement that is too broad	B	5

a. The seeds of the touch-me-not taste like black walnuts.

b. Plants use different methods for scattering their seeds.

c. The ocean carries coconut seeds great distances without harm.

d. Some seeds are scattered by popping, rolling or floating.

Total Comprehension Score
(Add your scores and enter the total on the graph on page 103.)

Categories of Comprehension Questions

No. 1: Subject Matter	No. 4: Clarifying Devices
No. 2: Supporting Details	No. 5: Vocabulary in Context
No. 3: Conclusion	No. 6: Main Idea

23. Temporary Tines

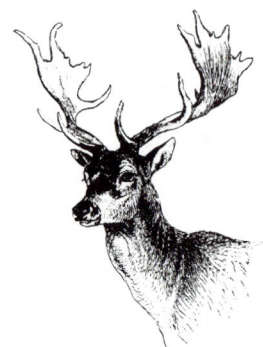

To all appearances, the antlers that adorn the heads of male members of the deer tribe seem to be as permanent as the animals themselves. They are, however, only a temporary addition. Each year they are shed and replaced with a new set.

Beginning in the spring as soft, swollen pads on the skull, they soon lengthen into clublike structures. While growing, they are covered with a fuzzy skin called *velvet*, beneath which blood circulates through a network of vessels. The tips are bulbous, and the entire antler is tender and easily damaged.

In two months they begin to show the general shape of the antlers to come. In some instances the growing antlers seem to be mere "spikes," while in others they appear to be elaborately branched. Four to six weeks later, they reach full size.

At full size, they undergo a surprising transformation. Beneath their furry covering the antlers harden and the blood supply stops. The velvet now dead and dry, peels off in strips, aided by the buck's vigorous rubbing against trees and bushes. The antlers are now bone-hard, with furrowed bases and pointed tines.

For a few weeks in autumn, they resist the incredible punishment of head-on, rutting-season clashes. Then one day, when the mating and fighting urge has passed, they suddenly drop from the buck's head, leaving only a pair of bony bases from which next year's set will grow.

The cycle is the same with deer, moose, elk, caribou — all of the deer family. Although the moose's huge palms may span seventy-six inches (about 193 centimeters) and weigh seventy pounds (about 31.8 kilograms) and the elk's majestic beams measure six feet or more (about 1.8 meters or more) in length, they nevertheless attain these impressive proportions in the short period of three or four months, making them the fastest growing animal tissue known.

What happens to the shed antlers? Within a few months they have usually been reduced to unrecognizable fragments by decay and the incisors of mice, squirrels and porcupines, to whom they are a welcome source of salt and calcium.

_____ **?** _____

	Possible Score	Your Score

1. This passage focuses mainly on the antlers of

　☐ a. deer.
　☐ b. moose.
　☐ c. elk.
　☐ d. caribou.

(15)　　○

2. How long does it usually take for a set of antlers to grow?

　☐ a. 1 month
　☐ b. 2 months
　☐ c. 3 to 4 months
　☐ d. 1 to 2 years

(15)　　○

3. We can conclude that antlers

　☐ a. are always soft and fuzzy.
　☐ b. are used in locating food.
　☐ c. are found only on the male.
　☐ d. grow at a very slow rate.

(15)　　○

4. The new antlers are covered with fuzzy skin called "velvet." How would they feel?

　☐ a. Soft
　☐ b. Harsh
　☐ c. Spiny
　☐ d. Moist

(15)　　○

5. The <u>rutting season</u> is the time for

　☐ a. seeking food.
　☐ b. leaving the den.
　☐ c. mating.
　☐ d. hibernating.

(15)　　○

6. Main Idea

	Answer	Score
Mark the main idea	M	10
Mark the statement that is a detail	D	5
Mark the statement that is too narrow	N	5
Mark the statement that is too broad	B	5

M a. Deer antlers are grown and shed anew each year.

   b. A deer's antlers only appear to be permanent.

   c. Antlers grow faster than any other animal tissue.

D d. Male deer antlers fall off after mating season.

Total Comprehension Score
(Add your scores and enter the total on the graph on page 103.)

Categories of Comprehension Questions

No. 1: Subject Matter	No. 4: Clarifying Devices
No. 2: Supporting Details	No. 5: Vocabulary in Context
No. 3: Conclusion	No. 6: Main Idea

92

24. Christmas Trees

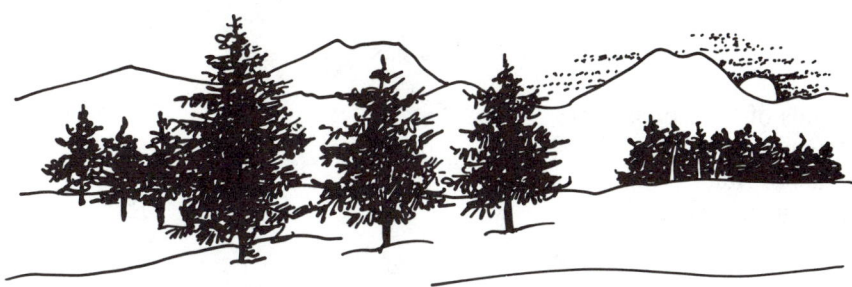

Purchasing live Christmas trees is a wonderful idea, but for people who have no place to plant them, regular Christmas trees are more practical. Using them doesn't actually endanger our forests because many Christmas trees are cultivated in special nurseries called *Christmas Tree Farms*. The trees on such farms are planted, fertilized, pruned and cut just for the holidays. Usually a tree such as you might purchase is four to six feet (about 1.2 to 1.8 meters) tall and is about ten years old. Because the trees have been specially grown, they are full and triangular shaped and ready to hold all your ornaments!

Most people believe a Christmas tree is a Christmas tree — and that no distinction is possible. But there are actually six different kinds of evergreens used for Christmas trees, not all of which are grown on farms. Some are young trees from forests that require thinning out to make additional growing room for existing trees.

The Scotch pine was imported from Europe long ago. It grows rapidly in dry, infertile soil and has become a beautiful bushy tree by the time it reaches your house.

The red pine is easily recognized by its reddish-brown bark. It grows straight and fast on many Christmas tree farms in the northeastern part of the United States.

The Douglas fir, which can grow to be nearly 300 feet (about 91.5 meters) tall, grows in the western part of the country on both sides of the Rocky Mountains.

Black spruce makes a fine, small table-top Christmas tree. These trees grow slowly in the marshes of the north. Besides being used at Christmas, these trees provide a sticky "resin" which is used in producing chewing gum and wood which is used in producing paper.

The balsam fir is very popular because its spicy odor brings the forest right indoors, and the needles remain on the tree for a long time after the presents are all unwrapped.

Eastern red cedars are really junipers that can grow about 100 feet (about 30.5 meters) tall. If the soil is really unproductive, though, the trees grow only to the size of a bush. The blue-gray berries have a clean, spicy fragrance if you crush them between your fingers.

No matter where your tree originated, it was probably grown especially for Christmas.

?

	Possible Score	Your Score

1. What would be another good title for this passage?

   ☐ a. Kinds of Christmas Trees
   ☐ b. How Much Is That Tree?
   ☐ c. Plastics Made from Trees
   ☐ d. Evergreens Never Die

   15 ◯

2. A Christmas tree which is 4–6 feet (about 1.2–1.8 meters) tall is about

   ☐ a. 2 years old.
   ☐ b. 5 years old.
   ☐ c. 8 years old.
   ☐ d. 10 years old.

   15 ◯

3. Because of Christmas tree farms,

   ☐ a. evergreens will probably never become extinct.
   ☐ b. more and more artificial trees are being bought.
   ☐ c. the price of Christmas trees has come down.
   ☐ d. many people refuse to buy real trees.

   15 ◯

4. The second paragraph tells us about

   ☐ a. Christmas tree farms.
   ☐ b. Scotch pines.
   ☐ c. artificial trees.
   ☐ d. tree ornaments.

   15 ◯

5. A <u>bushy</u> tree is

   ☐ a. sickly.
   ☐ b. small and thin.
   ☐ c. full and thick.
   ☐ d. very short.

   15 ◯

6. Main Idea

	Answer	Score
Mark the main idea	M	10
Mark the statement that is a detail	D	5
Mark the statement that is too narrow	N	5
Mark the statement that is too broad	B	5

a. The Scotch pine was imported from Europe.

b. A Christmas tree farm produces trees with full, triangular shapes.

c. Trees can be farmed just like other crops.

d. Most of the 6 kinds of Christmas trees are grown on farms.

Total Comprehension Score
(Add your scores and enter the total on the graph on page 103.)

Categories of Comprehension Questions

No. 1: Subject Matter	No. 4: Clarifying Devices
No. 2: Supporting Details	No. 5: Vocabulary in Context
No. 3: Conclusion	No. 6: Main Idea

25. The Bird That Survived

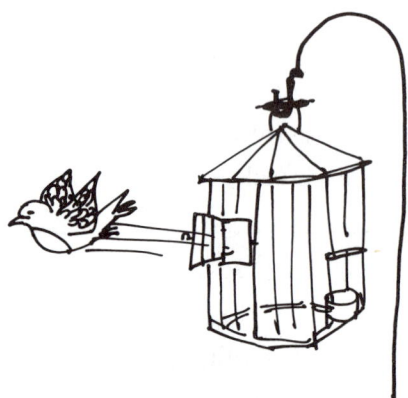

Animals removed from their natural environment to a foreign, wild environment are usually in trouble. But one brightly colored bird, the western linnet, or as some people call it, the *house finch*, survived this situation.

Around 1940, pet stores in New York City were selling western linnets in cages and labeling them "Hollywood Finches." They gave the birds this name because the linnets had been caught in California even though this violated the law. Wild birds may not be trapped and put in cages without special permission; even scientists must get this permission.

So that they wouldn't be discovered and fined, the shop managers secretly transported the linnets to far out on Long Island. As usual, some of the pet linnets escaped their owners for the outdoors. Normally, that would have been the end of these birds because they were not accustomed to the harsh winters, but it wasn't. They thrived and began to raise families.

Within a year or so, linnets had crossed Long Island Sound and were discovered in Connecticut, and soon they were sighted as far north as New Hampshire and as far south as North Carolina. You may even have seen some and not realized it.

The forehead, the sides of the head, and the neck and chest of adult males are a brilliant, cherry red, and there's also a reddish patch at the base of the tail. Females and young males resemble sparrows with grayish streaks on their abdomens and sides.

They are friendly birds and may become quite tame around humans. They are frequently the quickest to visit your bird feeder and the slowest to fly away when you approach.

House finches nest in different locations. Evergreen trees are favorite places, but underneath eaves and behind the shutters of barns and houses are also popular for nest building. Entangled vines clinging to a wall attract them for nesting, too. It's amazing how some birds can adapt to a new environment!

_____ **?** _____

	Possible Score	Your Score

1. This passage is about

   ☐ a. sparrows.
   ☐ b. cardinals.
   ☐ c. western linnets.
   ☐ d. blackbirds.

   15

2. House finches first came from

   ☐ a. California.
   ☐ b. New York City.
   ☐ c. Connecticut.
   ☐ d. North Carolina.

   15

3. When describing males and females, the writer suggests that

   ☐ a. the male is larger.
   ☐ b. the female is a dull color.
   ☐ c. the female is weaker.
   ☐ d. the male fights well.

   15

4. The female and young male finches look like

   ☐ a. crows.
   ☐ b. snow birds.
   ☐ c. sparrows.
   ☐ d. canaries.

   15

5. The opposite of a <u>foreign</u> environment is

   ☐ a. a natural environment.
   ☐ b. an artificial environment.
   ☐ c. a caged environment.
   ☐ d. the environment of a pet store.

   15

6. Main Idea

	Answer	Score
Mark the main idea	M	10
Mark the statement that is a detail	D	5
Mark the statement that is too narrow	N	5
Mark the statement that is too broad	B	5

a. Linnets can now be found from New Hampshire to North Carolina.

b. The law requires that you get a permit before caging a wild bird.

c. Sometimes a species will thrive when it is moved to a new area.

d. The western linnet survived a dramatic change in environment.

Total Comprehension Score
(Add your scores and enter the total on the graph on page 103.)

Categories of Comprehension Questions

No. 1: Subject Matter	No. 4: Clarifying Devices
No. 2: Supporting Details	No. 5: Vocabulary in Context
No. 3: Conclusion	No. 6: Main Idea

Acknowledgments

The passages appearing in this book have been reprinted with the kind permission of the following publications and publishers to whom the author is indebted:

Aramco World Magazine, published by The Arabian American Oil Company, New York, New York.

The Communicator, published by the New York State Outdoor Education Association, Syracuse, New York.

The Conservationist, published by the New York State Conservation Department, Albany, New York.

A Cornell Science Leaflet, published by the New York State College of Agriculture and Life Sciences, a unit of the State University, at Cornell University, Ithaca, New York.

Food, The Yearbook of Agriculture, published by the United States Department of Agriculture, Washington, D.C.

Handbook of Nature-Study, published by Comstock Publishing Company, Ithaca, New York.

Kansas Fish & Game, published by the Kansas Forestry, Fish and Game Commission, Pratt, Kansas.

National Wildlife, published by The National Wildlife Federation, Washington, D.C.

Outdoor Oklahoma, published by the Oklahoma Department of Wildlife Conservation, Oklahoma City, Oklahoma.

Pennsylvania Game News, published by the Pennsylvania Game Commission, Harrisburg, Pennsylvania.

Ranger Rick's Nature Magazine, published by The National Wildlife Federation, Washington, D.C.

The Tennessee Conservationist, published by the Tennessee Department of Conservation and the Tennessee Game and Fish Commission.

Answer Key: Book 13

Passage 1:	1.c	2.b	3.d	4.c	5.a	6a.N	6b.B	6c.M	6d.D
Passage 2:	1.c	2.b	3.b	4.c	5.d	6a.D	6b.B	6c.N	6d.M
Passage 3:	1.a	2.d	3.c	4.d	5.a	6a.B	6b.M	6c.N	6d.D
Passage 4:	1.a	2.b	3.d	4.b	5.d	6a.M	6b.B	6c.N	6d.D
Passage 5:	1.b	2.a	3.a	4.d	5.c	6a.D	6b.B	6c.M	6d.N
Passage 6:	1.d	2.a	3.b	4.b	5.d	6a.M	6b.N	6c.B	6d.D
Passage 7:	1.b	2.a	3.b	4.d	5.b	6a.M	6b.D	6c.B	6d.N
Passage 8:	1.a	2.d	3.a	4.c	5.b	6a.D	6b.N	6c.M	6d.B
Passage 9:	1.d	2.a	3.b	4.b	5.d	6a.D	6b.M	6c.B	6d.N
Passage 10:	1.a	2.c	3.d	4.b	5.c	6a.N	6b.B	6c.M	6d.D
Passage 11:	1.c	2.b	3.d	4.a	5.c	6a.D	6b.B	6c.M	6d.N
Passage 12:	1.a	2.d	3.b	4.a	5.d	6a.D	6b.B	6c.N	6d.M
Passage 13:	1.b	2.d	3.a	4.c	5.d	6a.B	6b.D	6c.N	6d.M

Answer Key: Book 13

Passage 14:	1.c	2.a	3.b	4.a	5.c	6a.N	6b.B	6c.D	6d.M
Passage 15:	1.b	2.d	3.a	4.c	5.a	6a.B	6b.D	6c.M	6d.N
Passage 16:	1.b	2.b	3.b	4.a	5.b	6a.D	6b.B	6c.N	6d.M
Passage 17:	1.a	2.d	3.d	4.b	5.a	6a.D	6b.N	6c.B	6d.M
Passage 18:	1.b	2.b	3.a	4.b	5.d	6a.D	6b.N	6c.M	6d.B
Passage 19:	1.a	2.b	3.d	4.b	5.b	6a.D	6b.M	6c.N	6d.B
Passage 20:	1.b	2.a	3.c	4.a	5.d	6a.M	6b.B	6c.N	6d.D
Passage 21:	1.b	2.b	3.a	4.a	5.c	6a.B	6b.D	6c.M	6d.N
Passage 22:	1.a	2.d	3.b	4.d	5.c	6a.D	6b.B	6c.N	6d.M
Passage 23:	1.a	2.c	3.c	4.a	5.c	6a.M	6b.B	6c.D	6d.N
Passage 24:	1.a	2.d	3.a	4.a	5.c	6a.D	6b.N	6c.B	6d.M
Passage 25:	1.c	2.a	3.b	4.c	5.a	6a.N	6b.D	6c.B	6d.M

Diagnostic Chart (For Student Correction)

Directions: Write your final answers in the *upper* part of the passage block. Then correct your answers using the Answer Key on pages 100 and 101. If your answer is correct, do not make any more marks in the block. If your answer is incorrect, write the letter of the correct answer in the *lower* part of the block.

Reading Passage

Categories of Comprehension Skills	1	2	3	4	5	6	7	8	9	10	11	12	13	14	15	16	17	18	19	20	21	22	23	24	25
1. Subject Matter																									
2. Supporting Details																									
3. Conclusion																									
4. Clarifying Devices																									
5. Vocabulary in Context																									
6. Main Idea — Main Idea																									
Detail																									
Too Narrow																									
Too Broad																									

Progress Graph

Directions: Write your Total Comprehension Score in the box under the number for each passage. Then put an *x* along the line above each box to show your Total Comprehension Score for that passage. Then make a graph of your progress. Draw a line to connect the *x*'s.

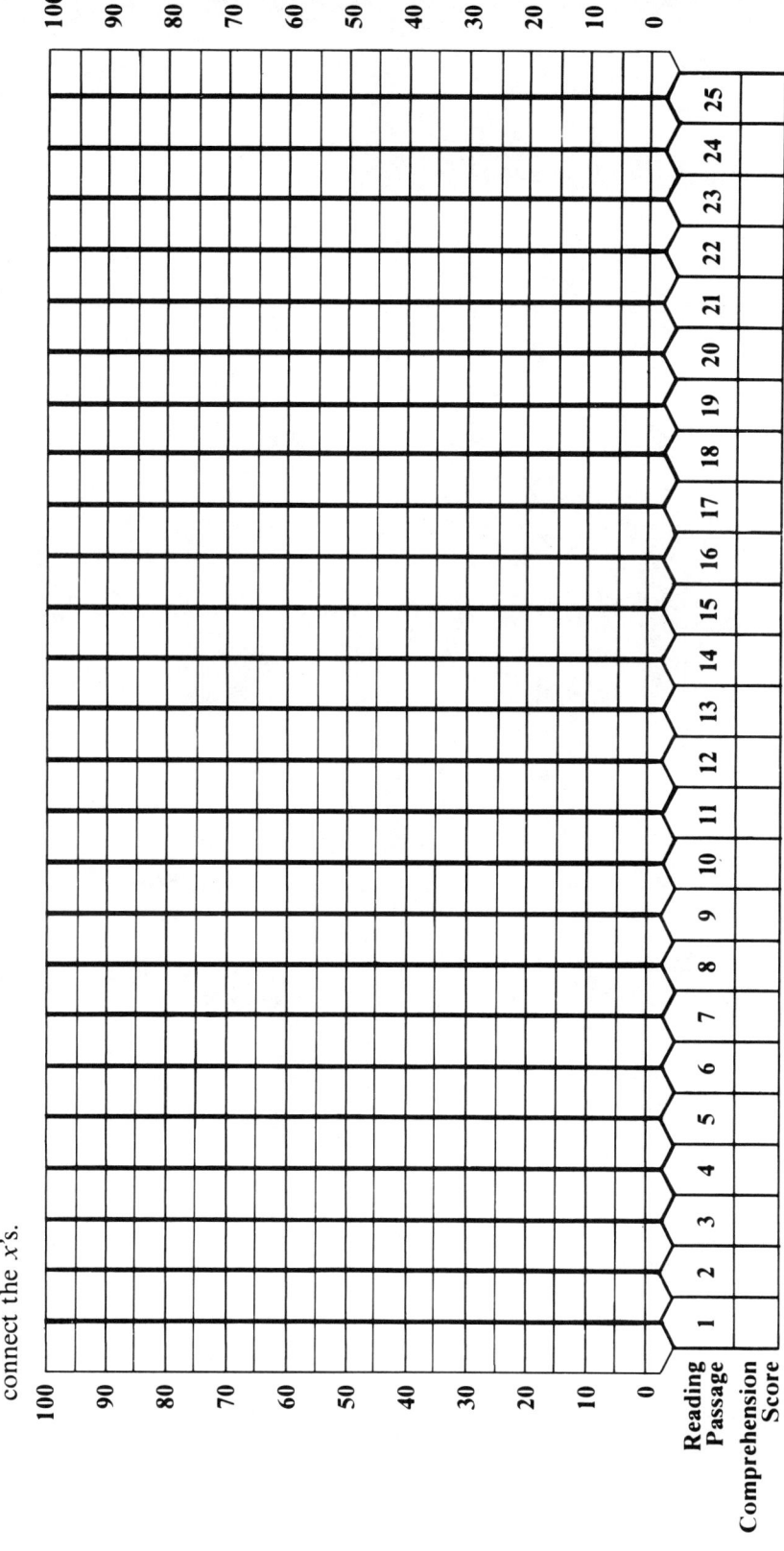

103

Classroom
Management
System

Essential Skills Series

Classroom Management System
(For Teacher Correction)

To the Teacher

The Classroom Management System provides an easy and effective way to individualize instruction. It can be used by reading specialists as well as by regular classroom teachers. The management system is designed to be equally effective when used with a single student, a small group, or a full-size class.

The Classroom Management System provides ongoing assessment of student work for both you and your student. It shows not only the amount of work completed, but also the quality of the work.

It serves as a diagnostic tool by revealing patterns of errors at a glance. For example, if a student has difficulty identifying subject matter (question #1 in each set of questions throughout the *Essential Skills Series*), a pattern of errors will appear in the Subject Matter column of the Classroom Management System Record Sheet. This will enable you to focus on the specific skills needs of each student.

The Classroom Management System Record Sheet is on pages 108-109. Both pages may be duplicated and stapled together.

How to Use the Classroom Management System Record Sheet

Step 1: Have the student answer the questions for each *Essential Skills* passage under the appropriate question heading.

Passage	① Subject Matter	② Supporting Details	③ Conclusion	④ Clarifying Devices	⑤ Vocabulary in Context	⑥ Main Idea				Number Correct	Errors Corrected
						a	b	c	d		
1	d	c	a	b	d			N D B M			

Step 2: Circle any incorrect answers and fill in the total number correct.

| 1 | d | ⓒ | a | b | d | | | (N) D B M | | 6 | |

Step 3: Have the student correct his or her incorrect answers.

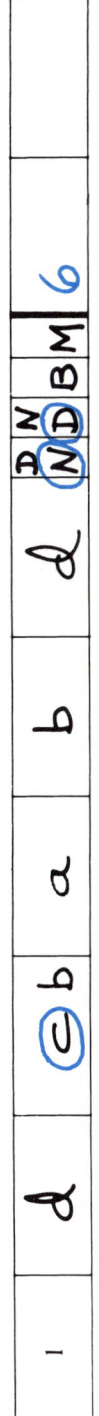

Step 4: Give assistance as needed and, if necessary, correct the student's adjusted answers.

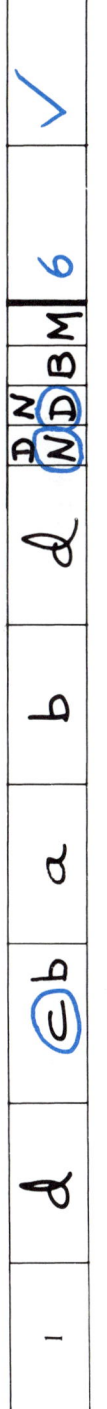

Step 5: Have the student go on to the next passage.

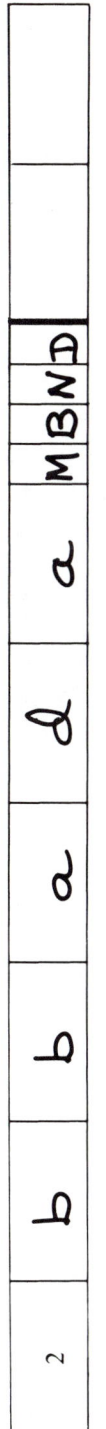

Step 6: Repeat Steps 1-4. If the class is large, it may be necessary to have students complete two or three passages before you correct them. This will slow the "traffic" at your desk.

Note: It is important for students to analyze and, to the extent possible, correct their own errors (Step 3).

107

Essential Skills Series

Classroom Management System Record Sheet
(For Teacher Correction)

Name _____
Teacher _____
Date _____
Book Number _____

To the Student: Write your answers in the spaces provided. (See the Example below.) Your teacher will circle any incorrect answers. Then go back over the questions and correct your mistakes.

Passage	① Subject Matter	② Supporting Details	③ Conclusion	④ Clarifying Devices	⑤ Vocabulary in Context	⑥ Main Idea a b c d	Number Correct	Errors Corrected
Example	c	(b) a	d	a	c	a (b) c B		
1								
2								
3								
4								
5								
6								
7								
8								
9								
10								

	①	②	③	④	⑤	⑥	
11							
12							
13							
14							
15							
16							
17							
18							
19							
20							
21							
22							
23							
24							
25							

This record sheet may be duplicated for classroom use by teachers. From *Essential Skills Series* by Walter Pauk, copyright © 1982 by Jamestown Publishers. Classroom Management System by Thomas F. Kelly, Ph.D.